# Clinical Cases in Dermatology

**Series Editor**
Robert A. Norman, Tampa, FL, USA

This series of concise practical guides is designed to facilitate the clinical decision-making process by reviewing a number of cases and defining the various diagnostic and management decisions open to clinicians.

Each title is illustrated and diverse in scope, enabling the reader to obtain relevant clinical information regarding both standard and unusual cases in a rapid, easy to digest format. Each focuses on one disease or patient group, and includes common cases to allow readers to know they are doing things right if they follow the case guidelines.

Nicholas Brownstone • Wilson Liao
Tina Bhutani
Editors

# Clinical Cases in Atopic Dermatitis

Springer

*Editors*
Nicholas Brownstone
Department of Dermatology
Temple University Hospital
Philadelphia, PA, USA

Wilson Liao
Department of Dermatology
University of California, San Francisco
San Francisco, CA, USA

Tina Bhutani
Psoriasis and Skin Treatment Center
University of California, San Francisco
San Francisco, CA, USA

ISSN 2730-6178 ISSN 2730-6186 (electronic)
Clinical Cases in Dermatology
ISBN 978-3-031-52146-1 ISBN 978-3-031-52147-8 (eBook)
https://doi.org/10.1007/978-3-031-52147-8



This Springer imprint is published by the registered company Springer Nature Switzerland AG
The registered company address is: Gewerbestrasse 11, 6330 Cham, Switzerland

Paper in this product is recyclable.

*NB—To Aunt Jean and Uncle Nick and to my mentors in dermatology: Tina Bhutani MD, Wilson Liao MD, John Koo MD, Mark Lebwohl MD, James Del Rosso DO, Darrell Rigel MD, Sylvia Hsu MD. Thank you for everything you have done for me.*

*TB—To my husband Glen and my two children, Kiaan and Haley. Thank you for your support and for being my shining lights!*

*WL—To Joule, Mei-Hwa, Hae-Won, and Ethan: thank you for your love and support.*

# Foreword

We are now squarely within "The Decade of Eczema": the explosion in understanding of atopic dermatitis has—finally!—led to new and better treatments unlike anything we have ever seen. These novel and more targeted treatments have paved the way for an even better understanding of the disease and have importantly highlighted the glaring gaps that remain. This process is what I have heard referred to as "the virtuous cycle of drug development." It represents that we have achieved critical mass, so to speak, and are now on a wonderful path.

Yet, the path is not without its perils. We have moved from a relatively simplistic view of eczema to one that recognizes a multifaceted interplay between genetic, environmental, and immunological factors. We see the pathogenic factors at play: the dysregulated immune responses, defective skin barrier function, dysbiosis of the microbiome, as well as the neuro-behavioral aspects of the disease. It is clear that this compelling narrative now requires a great deal of work towards successful translation into tangible, practical patient care.

*Clinical Cases in Atopic Dermatitis* emerges at a pivotal juncture in this journey, serving as a capstone of the collective advancements over recent years. However, it is more than just an update or a summary of the science, as it also reflects on the broader philosophy of medicine and has a clinician's eye for fusing these fragments of insight into a solid sculpture of wisdom.

For those seeking to navigate the rich landscape of novel biologic medications and JAK inhibitors that have emerged in recent years, this book will prove an invaluable guide. It carefully dissects the complex mechanisms of action of these treatments, illustrating their practical application with real-world clinical cases. In doing so, the abstract becomes concrete when rooted in these patient stories. This approach is a testament to the commitment to delivering not just evidence-based medicine, but also more empathetic and personalized care.

In this rapidly evolving field, *Clinical Cases in Atopic Dermatitis* serves as an essential resource for all those who deal with eczema, whether seasoned experts or trainees just beginning their journey. With luck, this book will enter into that virtuous cycle as well, improving patient care and inspiring clinicians to continue along the path as we push back against this terrible disease.

Department of Dermatology
Northwestern University,
Chicago, IL, USA

Peter Lio

# Preface

When we entered the profession of medicine, we all signed up to be "lifelong learners." The management of atopic dermatitis illustrates this point beautifully. For many decades, our understanding of the pathophysiology of atopic dermatitis was limited and treatment was restricted to topical corticosteroids and non-targeted oral immunosuppressive agents. In the last decade, a paradigm shift has occurred where we now have elucidated immunopathogenic mechanisms of atopic dermatitis down to specific cell types and cytokines.

Within the last 5 years, there has been a revolution in therapy with the FDA approval of multiple biologic medications and JAK inhibitors for atopic dermatitis. Furthermore, our understanding of the etiology, disease associations, and comorbidities of atopic dermatitis has expanded. Given this rapid change, new resources covering these topics are greatly needed.

This book seeks to address this need by covering the latest research on atopic dermatitis including key chapters on the newest FDA-approved therapies, updates on comorbidities, special considerations in skin of color, the role of diet and environment, impact on quality of life, pipeline therapies, and a review of atopic dermatitis spectrum disorder. We believe that practicing dermatologists, dermatology trainees, and medical students will all have something new to learn from this book.

The authors contributing to this book have outstanding expertise in the diagnosis and treatment of this disease. The topics they discuss will give the busy dermatology provider an excellent overview of the cutting-edge principles regarding the new therapies and concepts in management for atopic dermatitis in a fun, case-based format. If the knowledge you gain from reading this book helps even just one patient, we view that as a success!

Philadelphia, USA — Nicholas Brownstone
San Francisco, USA — Tina Bhutani
San Francisco, USA — Wilson Liao

# Acknowledgments

We would like to thank the patients with eczema who have taught us so much and inspired us to be better physicians.

# Contents

# Chapter 1
# Introduction to Atopic Dermatitis (AD)

**Gillian N. Kasper, McKenzie A. Dirr, Nicholas Brownstone, and John Koo**

**Case Title** A 29-year-old male presents with his 4-year-old daughter for a chief complaint of an "itchy rash" inside her elbows and behind her knees.

**Case**

It is your first patient after lunch, and you are seeing a 4-year-old female who complains of an "itchy rash" on the inside of her elbows and behind her knees. The patient is accompanied by her father. You observe an erythematous dermatitis with oozing and crusting on the flexural surfaces of the skin. The patient's father states that this has been present for the past few weeks; however, the only other medical condition the patient suffers from is asthma. You diagnose the patient with atopic dermatitis (AD) and ask the father if he has any questions. The father explains that he is currently in medical school and is interested in learning about the incidence, prevalence, pathophysiology, morphology, and histopathology of AD. How do you respond?

---

G. N. Kasper (✉)
Lewis Katz School of Medicine at Temple University, Philadelphia, PA, USA
e-mail: gillian.kasper@temple.edu

M. A. Dirr
Medical University of South Carolina College of Medicine, Charleston, SC, USA

N. Brownstone
Department of Dermatology, Temple University, Philadelphia, PA, USA

J. Koo
University of California, San Francisco, San Francisco, CA, USA



N. Brownstone et al. (eds.), *Clinical Cases in Atopic Dermatitis*, Clinical Cases in Dermatology, https://doi.org/10.1007/978-3-031-52147-8_1

**Board Review Question**
Which of the following is an essential feature that must be present when diagnosing atopic dermatitis?

A. Lichenification
B. Pruritus
C. Atopy
D. Xerosis
E. Early age of onset

Atopic dermatitis (AD) is a chronic relapsing inflammatory skin condition and is one of the most prevalent inflammatory skin diseases [1, 2]. It usually presents in childhood and can persist into adulthood [2]. The onset of disease is most common by 5 years of age [1]. The disorder is represented by a recurrent, pruritic, localized eczematous dermatitis that often presents with seasonal fluctuations [2]. Many of these patients who present with AD will also have asthma, allergic rhinitis, and/or food allergies [2]. The lesions are erythematous and characterized by papules, papulovesicles, edema, crusting, and scaling with possible hyperpigmentation or hypopigmentation after healing [2]. In infants, eczema may be more widespread and affect areas including the head, face, cheeks, arms, and legs; however, with increasing age, the lesions tend to be confined mainly to the flexural areas of the arms and legs [2]. Table 1.1 lists common locations of AD in different age groups. Pruritus is a hallmark of atopic dermatitis, which can induce excoriations, bleeding, and/or hemorrhagic crusts as well as eventual lichenification and, in some patients, formation of prurigo nodularis [2]. Patients who suffer from atopic dermatitis can also present with several other associated clinical signs including thinning or loss of the lateral eyebrows (Hertoghe's sign) and/or hyperlinear palms [2]. Atopic dermatitis has a chronic and fluctuating course, but other clinical signs including xerosis and lichenification persist between flares of disease [2]. Table 1.2 lists some

**Table 1.1** Common locations of atopic dermatitis based on age

| Age | Location of lesion |
|---|---|
| Infants | Face, scalp, cheeks, joints, extensor surfaces |
| Children | Flexural surfaces (elbows and knees), neck, ankles |
| Teens and adults | Hands, neck, flexural surfaces (elbows and knees), ankles, feet, skin around eyes |

**Table 1.2** Common features of atopic dermatitis

| |
|---|
| Erythematous lesion involving the flexural surfaces |
| Pruritus (essential) |
| Early age of onset |
| Atopy |
| Xerosis |
| Lichenification |
| Chronic and relapsing course |
| Family history |

common clinical features of atopic dermatitis that patients may present with. Chronic and relapsing atopic dermatitis can lead to decreased quality of life for patients and their families, so it is important to recognize and treat AD when applicable [2].

The incidence of AD has increased two to three fold since the 1970s with 15–20% of children and 1–3% of adults being affected worldwide [1]. The prevalence of AD in the United States is 11.3–12.7% in children and 6.9–7.6% in adults [3]. The highest incidence occurs between the ages of 3 and 6 months with the onset of disease commonly presenting by 5 years old [1]. Around 60% of patients will go on to develop AD during the first year of life and 90% during the first 5 years of life [1]. If children develop AD before 2 years of age, 20% of them will develop persisting symptoms of the disease [1]. AD most commonly resolves by adulthood; however, 10–30% of patients will continue to experience symptoms of AD [1]. AD has been shown to be more persistent in males, in patients who develop AD later in life, and in those who have severe cases of AD [1]. In 2010, it was estimated that around 230 million people, mostly those who are undiagnosed, are living with atopic dermatitis worldwide [4].

The pathophysiology of atopic dermatitis includes a permutation between a dysfunctional epidermal barrier, skin microbiome abnormalities, and a type 2-driven immune dysregulation [4]. An example of this interplay includes a patient who may have a filaggrin deficiency that causes a barrier weakness leading to inflammation and T-cell infiltration [4]. Infection or colonization with *Staphylococcus aureus* can damage the skin barrier and cause an inflammatory response [4]. A Th2 cell predominant response can also harm barrier function, can cause itching, and can contribute to dysbiosis [4]. Genetics play a strong role in the development of atopic dermatitis with a family history of AD being the strongest identifiable risk factor for developing the disease [4]. Filaggrin (FLG) null mutations contribute to impairing the skin barrier function and can increase the risk of developing AD [3]. Homozygous FLG mutations are related to an increased risk of severe AD associated with an earlier onset and longer persistence of symptoms as well as skin infections [3]. Regarding immune dysregulation, IL-4 and IL-13 (type 2 cytokines) have roles in skin barrier dysfunction, suppression of antimicrobial peptides (AMP), and allergic inflammation [3]. IL-17 and IL-22 have also been shown to be higher in patients with AD and are associated with skin barrier dysfunction [3].

Regarding the microbiome and dysbiosis, patients with AD have decreased skin bacterial diversity with increased *Staphylococcus* and *Corynebacterium* and decreased *Streptococcus*, *Propionibacterium, and Acinetobacter* during flares of AD [3]. Bacterial diversity was increased after treatment of AD [3]. There is a higher predominance of *S. aureus* in patients with more severe AD, and this has a significant role in the development and flares of AD [3]. Overall, there are multiple factors that contribute to the pathogenesis of atopic dermatitis including gene mutations, skin barrier dysfunction, immune dysregulation, and microbial dysbiosis.

Morphologic features that are characteristic for the diagnosis of AD include pruritic and eczematous plaques and papules that can present as acute, subacute, or chronic in nature [5]. Many patients will also have xerosis [5]. Acute lesions usually present as diffuse erythematous patches with oozing papulovesicles [5]. Subacute lesions usually present as red, dry, and scaly [5]. Chronic lesions are usually poorly demarcated and may present as scaly patches and plaques with excoriations and lichenification [5]. The lesions can affect nearly any part of the body but usually show some specific distributions that may differ based on the age of the patient [5]. In infants, atopic dermatitis is usually acute and normally presents with lesions on the face and the extensor surfaces of the limbs, and the trunk may also be affected [5, 6]. Starting around 1–2 years of age, polymorphous skin lesions are seen, which normally present in the flexural areas/folds [5]. Adolescents and adults normally present with lichenified and excoriated plaques at the flexural folds, wrists, ankles, and possibly eyelids; there is also a head and neck type, where the upper trunk, shoulders, and scalp can also be involved [5, 6]. Interestingly, adults may present with solely chronic hand eczema [5]. There is a morphological variant known as the follicular type, which can be characterized by densely aggregated follicular papules, which is commonly seen in dark-skinned patients [5]. There is also a morphological variant known as the prurigo type, which involves erythematous, sometimes excoriated papules and indurated nodules, which can be seen in patients with long-standing disease from chronic rubbing and scratching[5].

Regarding the histopathology of atopic dermatitis, the skin of patients with AD that clinically appears without current lesion contains a small amount of perivascular T-cell infiltration that suggests some minimal underlying inflammation [7]. Papular skin lesions that may develop in someone with acute onset AD show intercellular edema/spongiosis of the epidermis [7]. Acute skin lesions also show perivascular T-cell infiltration with monocyte macrophages in the dermis as well as eosinophils [7]. Chronic AD lesions that may be lichenified usually show a hyperplastic epidermis with elongation of the rete ridges, hyperkeratosis, and small amounts of spongiosis [7]. Overall, AD's histopathology is mainly represented by spongiosis and perivascular dermal infiltration of T cells and macrophages [8].

**Board Review Question Explanation**

What is an essential feature (must be present) to diagnose atopic dermatitis?

A. Lichenification
B. Pruritus (correct)
C. Atopy
D. Xerosis
E. Early age of onset

Explanation: Essential features that must be present to make the diagnosis of AD include pruritus and eczematous lesions that show typical morphology and have a chronic or relapsing history [5]. Atopy, xerosis, and early age of onset are common features that help support the diagnosis of AD but are not essential to the diagnosis [5]. Lichenification may present in chronic AD from recurrent itching, but it is not essential to diagnose AD especially in the acute setting [2].

**Key Takeaway Points**

- AD is one of the most common inflammatory skin diseases.
- AD commonly presents in childhood and can persist into adulthood.
- AD lesions are recurrent, pruritic, and erythematous and characteristically involve the flexural skin folds.
- AD pathophysiology includes a combination of dysfunctional epidermal barrier, skin microbiome dysbiosis, and immune dysregulation.
- AD's histopathological pattern is spongiotic dermatitis.
- AD is a "spectrum disease" with heterogeneous manifestations even in the same patient at different time points.

## References

1. Avena-Woods C. Overview of atopic dermatitis. AJMC. 2017;23:S115–23.
2. Ständer S. Atopic dermatitis. N Engl J Med. 2021;384(12):1136–43. https://doi.org/10.1056/nejmra2023911.
3. Kim J, Kim BE, Leung DY. Pathophysiology of atopic dermatitis: clinical implications. Allergy Asthma Proc. 2019;40(2):84–92. https://doi.org/10.2500/aap.2019.40.4202.
4. Langan SM, Irvine AD, Weidinger S. Atopic dermatitis. Lancet. 2020;396(10247):345–60. https://doi.org/10.1016/s0140-6736(20)31286-1.
5. Weidinger S, Novak N. Atopic dermatitis. Lancet. 2016;387(10023):1109–22. https://doi.org/10.1016/s0140-6736(15)00149-x.
6. Correale CE, Walker C, Murphy L, Craig TJ. Atopic dermatitis: a review of diagnosis and treatment. Am Fam Physician. 1999;60(4):1191–210.
7. Bieber T. Atopic dermatitis. Ann Dermatol. 2010;22(2):125–37. https://doi.org/10.5021/ad.2010.22.2.125.
8. Girolomoni G, de Bruin-Weller M, Aoki V, Kabashima K, Deleuran M, Puig L, Bansal A, Rossi AB. Nomenclature and clinical phenotypes of atopic dermatitis. Ther Advances Chronic Dis. 2021;12:204062232110029. https://doi.org/10.1177/20406223211002979.

# Chapter 2
# Atopic Dermatitis in Skin of Color

**Chiamaka Ohanenye, Danny Zakria, and Alexandra K. Golant**

**Case Title** A 16-year-old African American male presents with a chief complaint of a "dry, itchy rash."

**Case**

It's a cold, winter morning, and you see a 16-year-old African American male patient accompanied by his father who presents with a few months' history of a "dry, itchy rash." He is type V on the Fitzpatrick scale. The rash is dark purple and brown in hue, scaly, and lichenified and is located on the flexural surfaces of the arms, legs, and ankles. The patient's father complains that he has brought his son to two dermatologists prior to you, and neither was able to adequately manage his son's rash. His father is concerned that his child was misdiagnosed, which is delaying his son's treatment. On further clinical examination, you diagnose the patient with atopic dermatitis. The patient's father asked why the other dermatologists were unable to diagnose his son. How do you respond?

C. Ohanenye
Department of Dermatology, Temple University, Philadelphia, PA, USA
e-mail: amaka@temple.edu

D. Zakria (✉) · A. K. Golant
Department of Dermatology, Icahn School of Medicine at Mount Sinai, New York, NY, USA
e-mail: alexandra.golant@mountsinai.org



N. Brownstone et al. (eds.), *Clinical Cases in Atopic Dermatitis*, Clinical Cases in Dermatology, https://doi.org/10.1007/978-3-031-52147-8_2

**Board Review Question**
What type of filaggrin mutation is associated with increased prevalence of atopic dermatitis?

A. Gain-of-function mutation
B. Dominant-negative mutation
C. Loss-of-function mutation
D. Lethal mutation

## Main Text

Atopic dermatitis (AD) is a common inflammatory skin condition seen across the globe. It affects populations of all races and ethnicities. AD typically begins in early childhood, with 10% of children in the United States reported to have AD[1]. It is common for the disease to become less severe or resolve with advancing age. However, other patients have chronic AD that often persists into adulthood. In fact, 7% of American adults are reported to have AD[2]. Studies have shown that the prevalence and severity of AD can vary across different races and ethnicities in the United States. Data from the 2003 National Survey of Children's Health shows that the prevalence of AD in Black children is 15.9% and in White children is 9.7% in the United States [1]. Black children are 1.7 times more likely to develop AD than White children [2], and Black and Hispanic children are more likely to have persistent AD and more severe disease [3]. The epidemiologic inequalities of AD across races and ethnicities are nuanced and complex, but important when considering its treatment in SOC patients.

There are genetic mutations associated with AD that differ between ethnicities. Genome-wide association studies have been conducted that suggest that genes that are involved in the synthesis of epithelial barrier proteins and epithelial immune regulation are mutated at different rates, depending on race and ethnicity [4]. One of the genes indicated in these studies is the filaggrin gene, which encodes the filaggrin protein. Loss-of-function filaggrin mutations are associated with the development of AD. Filaggrin plays a significant role in the formation of the insoluble keratin matrix found in the stratum corneum [4]. This matrix provides stability to the outermost layer of the skin by providing a scaffold for lipids, thereby promoting water retention in the epidermis and homeostasis of the epidermis. Studies have shown that filaggrin loss-of-function mutations are seen in 50% of AD patients of European descent and 27% of AD patients of Asian descent. These studies also show that these mutations are six times less common in AD patients of African descent, even in those with severe AD [5]. These findings suggest that the filaggrin mutation plays less of a role in the pathogenesis of AD in certain SOC populations.

The ceramide content of the skin has also been shown to differ across races. Ceramides constitute the majority of lipids in the stratum corneum. These lipids play a role in retaining moisture and forming the permeability barrier of the skin.

Kitatani et al. found that SOC patients with AD tend to have deficiencies in both ceramide quantity and composition, which predispose them to the development of AD [6]. Multiple studies have shown that ceramide level and ceramide-to-cholesterol ratio are lowest in black skin [7, 8]. These studies also show that ceramide levels tend to be higher in White skin and highest in Asian skin.

AD is a heterogeneous condition with multiple factors that contribute to its prevalence and severity. It has been shown that SOC patients are more likely to have severe AD than White patients [9]. There are several explanations that may explain why patients of certain races tend to have more severe AD. These include delayed presentation due to decreased utilization of healthcare, delayed diagnosis, and environmental and socioeconomic factors, among others. For example, studies have shown that Black patients are less likely to see a provider regarding their AD than White patients [10]. Dermatologists and other healthcare providers should be cognizant of the genetic, psychosocial, and environmental differences that their SOC patients may present with when treating AD.

Many clinical features of AD are similar across races and ethnicities. Despite this, the clinical presentation of AD may vary depending on skin type (Table 2.1). The classic description of AD is dry, scaly, pruritic, and erythematous skin primarily seen on flexural surfaces of the body, such as the popliteal or antecubital fossae. These lesions can be complicated by the presence of exudate, fissuring, and crusting. This classic phenotype of AD is commonly taught and depicted in dermatology textbooks. However, in darker skin tones, AD often presents differently than what is seen in lighter skin types. Black, Hispanic, and Asian patients can have a more prominent perifollicular or papular morphology of their AD lesions than White patients [11]. Black and Asian patients with AD tend to have more lichenification than White patients. Black and Hispanic patients with AD tend to more frequently have truncal lesions [11]. AD in Black patients may present on extensor surfaces, which deviates from the classic presentation of AD. Dennie-Morgan lines and periorbital dark circles are more commonly seen in Black patients. This is likely due to increased pruritus and itching of the orbital area. Prurigo nodularis and hyperlinearity of palms are additional findings more commonly seen in Black patients with AD[12]. Some Asian patients with AD can have a more of a psoriasiform presentation with more well-demarcated lesions with scaling and increased epidermal hyperplasia[11].

Additionally, AD lesions on darker skin tones may not always appear erythematous. AD may present as a wide range of colors that some providers may not consider. Rather than being bright red, these lesions can appear violaceous, deep brown, or gray and may be nearly undetectable in certain skin types. The gestalt of using

**Table 2.1** Differences in presentation of AD across different ethnic groups

| |
|---|
| *Black:* Truncal lesions, perifollicular or papular morphology, Dennie-Morgan lines, lichenification, hyperlinearity of palms |
| *Asian:* Perifollicular or papular morphology, increased epidermal hyperplasia, clearer demarcation of lesions, lichenification |
| *Hispanic:* Truncal lesions, perifollicular or papular morphology |

erythema as a marker of disease in dermatologic conditions such as AD is fundamentally limiting. SOC can be pigmented to the point that it is incredibly difficult, if not impossible, to appreciate erythema. A keen eye that has studied and encountered erythema in dark skin may be able to recognize it and provide prompt and accurate diagnosis and care. However, some dermatologists may have limited experience diagnosing certain conditions in SOC patients. AD scoring systems like Scoring Atopic Dermatitis or Nottingham Eczema Severity Score were created to assess the clinical severity of AD and classify a patient's condition as mild, moderate, or severe. Erythema is one marker used to assess disease severity. While these scoring systems have their utility, they can result in misjudgment of the severity of AD in those with darker complexions [12], possibly leading to undertreatment of the disease.

There are apparent disparities in the diagnosis of AD across patients of different skin tones. Dermatologic disease can present less conspicuously in darker skin tones. If dermatologists are not properly trained in identifying pathology in SOC, diagnostic delay and undertreatment can occur. There are several reports in the literature that address how, in certain conditions, such as melanoma or drug reaction with eosinophilia and severe symptoms (DRESS) syndrome, SOC patients were inadequately treated, which led to the progression of the disease and a worse prognosis [13, 14]. These disparities in the diagnosis of AD in SOC patients can impact quality of life for those affected by this disease. Research from the University of Pennsylvania identified an association between race, AD, and absenteeism in school-aged children. Data from the Pediatric Eczema Elective Registry found that Hispanic and Black children were 3.4-fold and 1.5-fold more likely to miss over 6 days of school due to AD, respectively [15]. Although there are many factors that can contribute to these findings, this study suggests that AD may have a greater negative impact on the quality of life of SOC patients. Therefore, prompt and accurate diagnosis of AD is imperative in these populations.

Dermatology is a visual field. Because AD can appear markedly different than the description given or from images used in many textbooks and lectures, clinicians may have a more difficult time identifying AD in a patient with a darker skin tone. This can ultimately delay diagnosis and lead to the progression of a patient's condition. As a result, SOC patients are at higher risk of complications, such as permanent dyspigmentation and secondary infections. Providers may also underestimate disease severity because AD can look different in SOC and may be perceived as milder than it is. The ramifications of the disparity of AD diagnosis include decreased patient satisfaction and increased mistrust in the healthcare field.

There is a significant need for an improvement of care in SOC patients with AD. One approach is to increase the representation of AD in darker skin tones that are included in dermatologic resources such as textbooks, lectures, and search engine websites. Some dermatologists may not feel comfortable diagnosing skin conditions in darker skin types. In one study, nearly half of dermatologists and dermatology residents surveyed did not believe they had optimal training in identifying skin conditions in black skin [16]. Historically, pathology in SOC has not been taught as thoroughly as it should be in medical school and residency curriculums.

However, with diversity, equity, and inclusion initiatives, medical school and residency programs have made strides in correcting these gaps so that their graduates are equipped to treat any patient, regardless of their skin tone.

SOC patients can have added concerns with the dermatologic conditions they face due to their increased likelihood of residual persistent dyspigmentation. Post-inflammatory hyperpigmentation (PIH) is among the top 5 chief complaints in darker-skinned patients seen in dermatology clinics [17]. Therefore, another way of improving the care of AD in SOC patients is by being mindful of post-inflammatory dyspigmentation that can occur after an AD flare and treating it accordingly. Chronic inflammation from AD can lead to increased or decreased melanocyte deposition that may remain long after the flare subsides. This can lead to decreased quality of life from mental and physical ramifications of hypo- or hyperpigmentation. Dermatologists should be mindful of this when treating SOC patients with AD. Topical steroids are often the first-line treatment of AD; however, chronic use of these agents can cause steroid-induced pigmentary changes that may be more noticeable in those with darker skin tones. There are case reports that have shown that dupilumab can help improve PIH resulting from chronic AD. Other treatments of PIH include topical agents such as azelaic acid and hydroquinone, which inhibit tyrosinase and prevent melanin production. Agents such as aloe vera and niacinamide can also be employed to soothe areas of inflammation that predispose patients to PIH. Sun protection is also recommended to prevent further exacerbation of PIH.

Increasing the diversity of patients in clinical trials for AD is another way to improve care in this subset of patients. Despite having a higher prevalence of AD than White patients, SOC patients are often underrepresented in clinical trials. Sixty-two percent of participants in AD clinical trials conducted between 2000 and 2009 were identified as White. Eighteen percent were identified as Black, 7% identified as Asian, 2% identified as Hispanic, and 0.02% identified as Native American [18]. While some SOC populations are represented well in AD clinical trials, others are markedly underrepresented. Remedying this concern will ultimately provide valuable information on the applicability of study findings to diverse patient populations.

**Board Review Question Explanation**

What type of filaggrin mutation is associated with increased prevalence of atopic dermatitis?

A. Gain-of-function mutation
B. Suppressor mutation
C. Loss-of-function mutation (correct)
D. Lethal mutation

Explanation – Filaggrin is a component of the stratum corneum and a part of the skin barrier. It also helps maintain the pH of the skin. Loss-of-function mutations predispose individuals to genetic susceptibility to atopic dermatitis (reference: O'Regan GM, Sandilands A, McLean WHI, Irvine AD. Filaggrin in atopic dermatitis. J Allergy Clin Immunol. 2008 Oct;122(4):689–693. doi: 10.1016/j.jaci.2008.08.002. Epub 2008 Sep 5. PMID: 18774165).

**Key Takeaway Points**

- AD is an inflammatory skin disorder seen in all races and ethnicities.
- SOC patients often present with more severe disease, due to a variety of reasons.
- Genetic variability between races and ethnicities are present, which may partially explain differences in prevalence and severity across races and ethnicities.
- Greater representation of SOC patients in educational resources and clinical trials may help providers better understand and care for AD in this diverse population.

## References

1. Shaw TE, Currie GP, Koudelka CW, Simpson EL. Eczema prevalence in the United States: data from the 2003 National Survey of Children's health. J Invest Dermatol. 2011;131(1):67–73. https://doi.org/10.1038/jid.2010.251.
2. Martinez A, de la Rosa R, Mujahid M, Thakur N. Structural racism and its pathways to asthma and atopic dermatitis. J Allergy Clin Immunol. 2021;148(5):1112–20. https://doi.org/10.1016/j.jaci.2021.09.020.
3. Chung J, Simpson EL. The socioeconomics of atopic dermatitis. Ann Allergy Asthma Immunol. 2019;122(4):360–6. https://doi.org/10.1016/j.anai.2018.12.017.
4. Sandilands A, Sutherland C, Irvine AD, McLean WH. Filaggrin in the frontline: role in skin barrier function and disease. J Cell Sci. 2009;122(Pt 9):1285–94. https://doi.org/10.1242/jcs.033969.
5. Brunner PM, Guttman-Yassky E. Racial differences in atopic dermatitis. Ann Allergy Asthma Immunol. 2019;122(5):449–55. https://doi.org/10.1016/j.anai.2018.11.015.
6. Ohnishi Y, Okino N, Ito M, Imayama S. Ceramidase activity in bacterial skin flora as a possible cause of ceramide deficiency in atopic dermatitis. Clin Diagn Lab Immunol. 1999;6(1):101–4. https://doi.org/10.1128/CDLI.6.1.101-104.1999.
7. Wan DC, Wong VW, Longaker MT, Yang GP, Wei FC. Moisturizing different racial skin types. J Clin Aesthet Dermatol. 2014;7(6):25–32.
8. Jungersted JM, Høgh JK, Hellgren LI, Jemec GB, Agner T. Ethnicity and stratum corneum ceramides. Br J Dermatol. 2010;163(6):1169–73. https://doi.org/10.1111/j.1365-2133.2010.10080.x.
9. Ben-Gashir MA, Hay RJ. Reliance on erythema scores may mask severe atopic dermatitis in black children compared with their white counterparts. Br J Dermatol. 2002 Nov;147(5):920–5. https://doi.org/10.1046/j.1365-2133.2002.04965.x.
10. Fischer AH, Shin DB, Margolis DJ, Takeshita J. Racial and ethnic differences in health care utilization for childhood eczema: an analysis of the 2001-2013 medical expenditure panel surveys. J Am Acad Dermatol. 2017 Dec;77(6):1060–7. https://doi.org/10.1016/j.jaad.2017.08.035.
11. McKenzie S, Brown-Korsah JB, Syder NC, Omar D, Taylor SC, Elbuluk N. Variations in genetics, biology, and phenotype of cutaneous disorders in skin of color. Part II: differences in clinical presentation and disparities in cutaneous disorders in skin of color. J Am Acad Dermatol. 2022;87(6):1261–70. https://doi.org/10.1016/j.jaad.2022.03.067.
12. Kaufman BP, Guttman-Yassky E, Alexis AF. Atopic dermatitis in diverse racial and ethnic groups—variations in epidemiology, genetics, clinical presentation and treatment. Exp Dermatol. 2018;27:340–57. https://doi.org/10.1111/exd.13514.
13. Bean, E. L., Lewis, D. J., Weir, M. A., & Micheletti, R. G. (2023). Delayed diagnosis of DRESS syndrome in a patient with skin of color. Dermatol Online J, 29(1). doi:https://doi.org/10.5070/d329160221.

14. Gupta AK, Bharadwaj M, Mehrotra R. Skin cancer concerns in people of color: risk factors and prevention. Asian Pac J Cancer Prev. 2016;17(12):5257–64. https://doi.org/10.22034/APJCP.2016.17.12.5257.
15. Wan J, Margolis DJ, Mitra N, Hoffstad OJ, Takeshita J. Racial and ethnic differences in atopic dermatitis-related school absences among US children. JAMA Dermatol. 2019;155(8):973–5. https://doi.org/10.1001/jamadermatol.2019.0597.
16. Buster KJ, Stevens EI, Elmets CA. Dermatologic health disparities. Dermatol Clin. 2012;30(1):53–9., viii. https://doi.org/10.1016/j.det.2011.08.002.
17. Grayson C, Heath CR. Dupilumab improves atopic dermatitis and post-inflammatory hyperpigmentation in patient with skin of color. J Drugs Dermatol. 2020;19(7):776–8. https://doi.org/10.36849/JDD.2020.4937.
18. Hirano SA, Murray SB, Harvey VM. Reporting, representation, and subgroup analysis of race and ethnicity in published clinical trials of atopic dermatitis in the United States between 2000 and 2009. Pediatr Dermatol. 2012;29:749–55. https://doi.org/10.1111/j.1525-1470.2012.01797.x.

# Chapter 3
# Atopic Dermatitis and Internal Vessel Inflammation

**Amanda Loesch, Danny Zakria, and Alexandra K. Golant**

**Case Title** A 70-year-old female with a history of severe atopic dermatitis presents after a recent myocardial infarction (MI).

**Case**

It's a Friday afternoon in clinic. You are running late, but fortunately your final appointment is a longtime patient following up for her chronic condition. She is a 70-year-old female with a past medical history of severe atopic dermatitis. Her disease has been poorly controlled with topical treatment; however, she has never wished to escalate her care. The patient is visibly upset on exam and describes a recent hospitalization for a myocardial infarction (MI). She cannot understand why she had one – she doesn't drink alcohol or smoke cigarettes, and she maintains a healthy diet. She has no family history of heart attack or stroke. She asks if her skin condition could have had any role in causing her MI. How do you respond?

**Board Review Question**

Dysregulation of what immune pathway is most strongly associated with atopic dermatitis?

A. Th1
B. Th2
C. Th17
D. Th22
E. Treg

A. Loesch
Department of Dermatology, Temple University, Philadelphia, PA, USA
e-mail: Amanda.loesch@temple.edu

D. Zakria (✉) · A. K. Golant
Department of Dermatology, Icahn School of Medicine at Mount Sinai, New York, NY, USA
e-mail: alexandra.golant@mountsinai.org



N. Brownstone et al. (eds.), *Clinical Cases in Atopic Dermatitis*, Clinical Cases in Dermatology, https://doi.org/10.1007/978-3-031-52147-8_3

## Main Text

Atopic dermatitis (AD) has been associated with an increased risk of vascular inflammation, cardiovascular disease, and stroke. Recent literature has attributed this relationship to elevated levels of systemic inflammation, independent from genetic predisposition or other risk factors. A similar correlation has been established between psoriasis and internal vessel inflammation [1–7]. However, psoriasis and atherosclerosis are both Th1-mediated diseases, while AD is predominantly Th2-mediated.

A landmark study by Ungar et al. in 2020 showed a significant finding for vascular inflammation in patients with moderate-to-severe AD. The study used $^{18}$fluorodeoxyglucose-positron emission tomography/magnetic resonance imaging ($^{18}$F-FDG-PET/MRI) to determine the degree of vascular inflammation in 27 patients with moderate-to-severe AD versus 12 healthy controls without AD [8]. Similar imaging modalities have been used to demonstrate not only increased vascular inflammation in psoriasis but also the reduction of vessel inflammation with anti-inflammatory treatments [9]. Using this imaging modality, Ungar et al. identified a statistically significant elevation in inflammation of the right carotid arteries in patients with AD versus controls. Vessel inflammation of the aorta was also heightened in patients with AD approaching statistical significance. Additionally, the clinical severity of AD was associated with the degree of right carotid and aortic inflammation as well as increased C-reactive protein (CRP) [8]. CRP is a known nonspecific indicator of inflammation, often used as a biomarker for atherosclerosis and a prognostic tool in predicting cardiovascular events [10]. An established relationship between CRP and psoriasis disease severity exists [11]. CRP has previously been found to be elevated in moderate-to-severe AD, and the findings from Ungar et al. further support this relationship and the systemic nature of AD [12]. A valuable future study could use $^{18}$F-FDG-PET/MRI to assess the reversibility of vascular inflammation in patients with AD treated with systemic anti-inflammatory agents, similar to the previously mentioned experiment conducted for psoriasis [9].

A study by Villani et al. published in 2020 used a similar modality to evaluate vascular inflammation in patients with AD. In this study, 18F-FDG-PET/CT of the ascending aorta was used in parallel with skin and blood immune profiles and circulating microparticles to establish the effects of AD on vessel inflammation. Overall, study findings suggest that vascular inflammation in AD is associated with an enhanced Th2 response and clinical severity [13]. In this study, blood samples and punch biopsies were taken from both lesional and non-lesional skin in 30 patients with atopic dermatitis. Dysregulated genes were found in both lesional and non-lesional AD skin when compared to controls ($n$ = 26). The dysregulated genes included those related to T-cell activation and Th2 and Th17/Th22 pathways. Dysregulation of genes associated with a pro-atherosclerotic state was also found in both lesional and non-lesional AD skin samples. Patients with AD had higher amounts of Th2- and Th22-related markers in their circulation compared to healthy controls. The presence of skin immune markers in the blood suggests an interaction between these tissues in systemic inflammation in AD. These findings support the theory that the chronic inflammatory process that occurs in AD may predispose patients to cardiovascular disease.

Although controversial, atherosclerosis has been thought to predominantly be a Th1-mediated disease [14]. However, the findings from Villani et al. support previous discussions that Th2-mediated pathways may be associated with vascular inflammation [13, 15]. Specifically, the Th2 immune response likely prevails in the development of atherosclerosis in patients with AD [13]. Hjuler et al. conducted a study using cardiac computed tomography angiography (CCTA) to determine the coronary artery calcium score in patients with psoriasis and AD. Plaques were found in 38.2% of psoriasis patients ($n = 58$), 48.1% of AD patients ($n = 31$), and 21.2% of controls ($n = 33$). Psoriasis was associated with significant coronary stenosis, whereas AD was associated with milder vascular disease [16]. Typically, atherosclerosis is not known to be a result of Th2-mediated diseases such as atopic dermatitis. However, atopic dermatitis is thought to result from a complex interplay between Th2, Th17/Th22, Treg, and Th1 pathways. Th1 pathways are likely important during the chronic phase of AD, suggesting that chronic AD could contribute to the development of atherosclerosis [17]. Therefore, patients with chronic AD may benefit from systemic treatment to avoid cardiovascular risk factors [16].

Villani et al. also found higher levels of circulating endothelial microparticles in patients with AD, which correlated to vascular inflammation on 18F-FDG-PET/CT. Microparticles have been found to be associated with subclinical atherosclerosis and cardiovascular risk [18]. They are released by endothelial cells (EMPs) and platelets (PMPs) [19]. Microparticles are found to be increased in inflammatory diseases, such as psoriasis, as well as cardiovascular disease and metabolic syndrome [20]. Villani et al. saw a significant elevation of EMPs in AD compared to controls and higher levels of microparticles in patients with severe AD [13]. The correlation suggests that patients with AD may be at higher risk for atherosclerosis and other cardiovascular events secondary to a systemic inflammatory process.

Villani et al. also demonstrated that systemic treatment with dupilumab significantly reduced expression of atherosclerosis-related genes in AD [13]. Dupilumab is a biologic that inhibits IL-4R$\alpha$, therefore blocking IL-4 and IL-13, and is approved for the treatment of moderate-to-severe AD. This finding indicates that systemic treatment of moderate-to-severe AD may not only improve cutaneous disease but also may reduce systemic inflammation and the associated sequelae. Future studies should utilize 18F-FDG-PET/CT or MRI to evaluate a possible decrease in vascular inflammation with systemic intervention.

The association between AD and the dysregulation of pro-atherosclerotic genes is further supported by a study conducted by Pavel et al. that analyzed the proteomic skin profile in patients with moderate-to-severe AD in comparison to the blood proteome. Punch biopsies were obtained from lesional and non-lesional AD skin ($n = 20$), as well as healthy skin ($n = 28$). The patients in the AD subset abstained from topical treatment for a minimum of 2 weeks and systemic therapy for at least 4 weeks prior to biopsy. The analysis identified 161 differentially expressed proteins (DEP) in lesional AD skin and 69 DEPs associated with non-lesional AD skin. Upregulated proteins include those of inflammatory cells, such as dendritic cells, Th1, Th2, and Th17/Th22. The most significantly upregulated proteins were related to atherosclerosis and cardiovascular risk factors, such as E-selectin, matrix metalloproteinases (MMP), and platelet growth factor (PGF), as well as relevant cytokines and receptors, such as IL-6R and IL-8. These findings indicate that patients with AD harbor significant upregulation of atherosclerosis-inducing proteins even in non-lesional skin when compared to patients without AD, reflecting the systemic nature of inflammation in this disease [21]. Only 20 DEPs existed in blood, and out of those 20, 17 overlapped with those in AD skin. The overlapping proteins were those associated with Th2, Th1, Th17, MMP12, and IL-1RN. Expressions of atherosclerosis-associated markers FABP4, SORT1, and HMOX1 were seen in the blood of patients with AD [22, 23]. Since the protein expression in AD was significantly higher in the skin than the blood, it is postulated that the skin is the source of the upregulated proteins, as opposed to the blood. Further support for this phenomenon lies in the significant correlation found between expression of mRNA and protein in lesional AD, suggesting the translation of proteins in affected skin. Nonetheless, these findings corroborate the systemic nature of inflammation in patients with AD. Table 3.1 reviews the dysregulated factors in AD [21].

Angiogenesis is a process known to be associated with inflammation. The pathogenesis of psoriasis is related to the upregulation of vascular endothelial growth factor (VEGF), angiopoietins, and other markers of the angiogenesis process [24]. It is postulated that angiogenesis may play a role in systemic inflammation in AD as well. The histopathology findings of AD include edema of the intracellular epidermis and prominent infiltration of lymphocytes, dendritic cells, and monocytes into the perivascular dermis. In the acute setting, eosinophils may infiltrate into the perivascular dermis, while subacute and chronic findings include epidermal hyperkeratosis, acanthosis, and papillomatosis. Angiogenesis is required for all of these changes seen on histology [24]. Additionally, VEGF is elevated in the stratum corneum of lesional skin in AD and blood and correlates with disease severity [25, 26]. VEGF is released from endothelial cells, fibroblasts, and smooth muscle cells and activates angiogenesis in the skin. A study by Samochocki et al. evaluated the levels of VEGF and other cytokines in 83 patients with AD versus 25 controls [25]. They found elevated VEGF concentrations in the serum of patients with AD. Additionally, VEGF concentration was positively correlated with AD severity. Elevated blood levels of VEGF may correlate with leakage from keratinocytes in affected skin. Once in the blood, the increased inflammatory markers may act systemically to induce vascular changes [24, 25].

The pro-inflammatory state associated with AD may also increase the risk of stroke in patients with the disease. A population-based study in Taiwan identified AD as an independent risk factor for ischemic stroke. Su et al. followed 20,323 patients with AD and 20,322 healthy controls for up to 4 years to determine incidence of stroke and other cardiovascular events. Findings include a 33% increase in stroke in patients with AD and incidence correlated with disease severity [4]. The increased risk of stroke is likely due to systemic inflammation that promotes

**Table 3.1** Dysregulated factors in AD

| Category | Dysregulated factors | Effect on patients with AD |
|---|---|---|
| Microparticles | PMPs | Elevated in plasma |
| Microparticles | Annexin V+ | Elevated in plasma |
| Microparticles | EMPs (CD31, CD62+) | Elevated in plasma |
| Immune genes | T-cell activation (CD69, ICOS) | Dysregulated in lesional and non-lesional AD skin |
| Immune genes | Th2 (IL-4R, IL-13, IL-10, CCL13, CCL17, CCL18, CCL26) | Dysregulated in lesional and non-lesional AD skin |
| Immune genes | Th17/22 (IL-22, P13, S100A7/8/9/12) | Dysregulated in lesional and non-lesional AD skin |
| Atherosclerotic/ cardiovascular risk genes | S100A8, S100A9, S100A12, IL-36A, IL-36G | Dysregulated in lesional and non-lesional AD skin |
| Atherosclerotic/ cardiovascular risk genes | IL-6 | Dysregulated in lesioned skin |
| Protective factor for atherosclerosis | IL-37 | Downregulated in lesioned skin |
| Inflammatory cytokines | IL-36G/A/RN, IL-8 | Upregulated in lesional and non-lesional skin |
| Monocyte recruitment | CCL2 | Upregulated in lesional and non-lesional skin |
| Tissue remodeling | MMP1/12 | Upregulated in lesional and non-lesional skin |
| Atherosclerotic/ cardiovascular risk genes | Th22 (S100A8) | Upregulated in lesional and non-lesional skin |
| Inflammation and vascular adhesion | IL-6, ICAM1, SELE | Upregulated in lesioned skin |
| T-cell migration | CCL19/CCL21 | Upregulated in lesional and non-lesional skin |
| Immune genes | Th1 (IFN-γ) | Upregulated in lesional and non-lesional skin |
| Immune genes | Th17 (IL-17A, CL20, P13) | Upregulated in lesional and non-lesional skin |
| Epidermal hyperplasia | K16 | Upregulated in lesional and non-lesional skin |
| Inflammatory proteins | Th2 (IL-13, CCL13/CCL17/ CCL22/CCL26) | Upregulated in serum |
| Inflammatory proteins | Th1 (CXCL10) | Upregulated in serum |
| Inflammatory proteins | Th22 (IL-22, S100A8/A8) | Upregulated in serum |
| Innate immune markers | IL-8/CXCL8 | Undetectable in serum |

atherosclerosis, activation of the coagulation cascade, and thrombus formation. Etiology may stem from enhanced platelet activation and dysregulated fibrinolysis, leading to dense fibrin clots [27–29].

As increasing evidence suggests a link between AD and vascular inflammation, it is important to consider how lifestyle factors may contribute to these effects. A report of two population-based studies in US adults with AD concluded that patients with AD were more likely to have ever smoked, consume moderate to heavy amounts of alcohol, and have a higher BMI, lower rate of vigorous activity, increased odds of hypertension, increased odds of prediabetes, and sleep disturbances [3]. The direction of the correlations between alcohol use and smoking and AD remains to be elucidated. Sedentary lifestyle may prevail in patients with AD because sweat can sometimes trigger a flare, and therefore, patients may avoid exercise and vigorous activity, which may lead to weight gain, hypertension, and diabetes. However, when lifestyle factors were controlled for in multivariable models, the associations between AD and obesity, hypertension, and prediabetes prevailed, indicating that AD poses an additional risk [1, 3]. A case-control study by Silverberg et al. determined that moderate-to-severe AD in pediatric populations may be associated with increased systolic blood pressure (AD $n$ = 132, control $n$ = 143). More specifically, severe AD was associated with a systolic blood pressure of at least the 90th percentile, controlling for other risk factors. Therefore, screening of blood pressure in pediatric patients with AD may be a useful practice [6]. Nonetheless, targeting behavioral modifications is important in reducing any additional risk factors [1].

A population study that examined the effect of AD on adverse cardiovascular outcomes determined that after adjusting for confounding variables, MI, ischemic stroke, cardiovascular death, and major adverse cardiac events (MACEs) were reduced in patients with mild AD ($n$ = 26,898) but were increased in patients with severe AD ($n$ = 2527) on systemic therapy (control $n$ = 145,372) [2]. The authors believe these differences may be attributed to behavioral modifications, in that patients with greater access to healthcare who are compliant with treatment recommendations may have better disease control and thus never progress to severe AD. Therefore, these patients do not develop systemic manifestations of the disease [2]. Another study by Standl et al. similarly showed a lack of correlation between AD and cardiovascular events. Findings in this study indicated only a slight increase in angina pectoris (AP), hypertension, and peripheral artery disease (PAD) in patients with severe AD, likely due to their pro-inflammatory status [5]. Associations between AD and cardiovascular disease are not consistent throughout the literature and may occur in an unknown subset of patients. Therefore, it is not warranted to screen broadly without first elucidating the contribution of other risk factors such as smoking, alcohol, and physical activity [3].

Primary care physicians should be cognizant of the potential association of AD and a pro-inflammatory state. In patients with AD, screening for additional risk factors for cardiovascular disease including hypertension, metabolic syndrome, and stroke should be done regularly. Encouraging behavioral changes to decrease cumulative risk of vascular disease is prudent. The risk for relative increases in systolic blood pressure should be acknowledged in pediatric populations, and it is reasonable to screen patients with regular blood pressure monitoring. Overall, a systemic inflammatory state appears to be correlated with chronic, untreated, and/or severe AD. Thus, treatment with systemic anti-inflammatory medications should be considered in appropriate candidates to both improve cutaneous disease and decrease the sequelae of systemic inflammation.

**Board Review Question Explanation**

Which immune pathway is most prevalent in acute atopic dermatitis?

A. Th1
B. Th2 (correct)
C. Th17
D. Th22
E. Treg

Explanation: AD is thought to be predominately a Th2-mediated process, especially in the acute setting. Elevated levels of eosinophils and IgE are found in the serum of patients with AD, as well as increased skin expression of Th2 cytokines (IL-4, IL-5, and IL-13). IFN-γ, which is predominately seen in the Th1 pathway, is not elevated in acute AD. However, as AD lesions become more chronic, the expression of Th1 cytokines, such as IFN-γ and IL-12, becomes more pronounced [30].

**Key Takeaway Points**

- AD is a pro-inflammatory state that increases risk for stroke, cardiovascular disease, and systemic inflammation.
- Moderate-to-severe AD poses a greater risk for vascular inflammation than milder disease.
- AD causes increased angiogenesis, which leads to inflammation.
- AD is predominately a Th2-mediated process in the acute setting, but in chronic disease, the Th1 pathway predominates, leading to atherosclerosis.
- Behavioral risk factors, such as sedentary lifestyle, cigarette smoking, and alcohol use, can worsen cardiovascular and stroke risk in AD.
- AD may cause relatively elevated blood pressure in pediatric population.

## References


1. Silverberg JI, Greenland P. Eczema and cardiovascular risk factors in 2 US adult population studies. J Allergy Clin Immunol. 2015;135(3):721–8.e6. https://doi.org/10.1016/j.jaci.2014.11.023.
2. Andersen YMF, Egeberg A, Gislason GH, Hansen PR, Skov L, Thyssen JP. Risk of myocardial infarction, ischemic stroke, and cardiovascular death in patients with atopic dermatitis. J Allergy Clin Immunol. 2016;138(1):310–312.e3. https://doi.org/10.1016/j.jaci.2016.01.015.
3. Silverberg JI. Association between adult atopic dermatitis, cardiovascular disease, and increased heart attacks in three population-based studies. Allergy. 2015;70(10):1300–8. https://doi.org/10.1111/all.12685.
4. Su VY, Chen TJ, Yeh CM, Chou KT, Hung MH, Chu SY, Su KC, Chang YS, Lin YH, Liu CJ. Atopic dermatitis and risk of ischemic stroke: a nationwide population-based study. Ann Med. 2014;46(2):84–9. https://doi.org/10.3109/07853890.2013.870018.
5. Standl M, Tesch F, Baurecht H, Rodríguez E, Müller-Nurasyid M, Gieger C, Peters A, Wang-Sattler R, Prehn C, Adamski J, Kronenberg F, Schulz H, Koletzko S, Schikowski T, von Berg A, Lehmann I, Berdel D, Heinrich J, Schmitt J, Weidinger S. Association of Atopic Dermatitis with cardiovascular risk factors and diseases. J Invest Dermatol. 2017;137(5):1074–81. https://doi.org/10.1016/j.jid.2016.11.031.

6. Silverberg JI, Becker L, Kwasny M, Menter A, Cordoro KM, Paller AS. Central obesity and high blood pressure in pediatric patients with atopic dermatitis. JAMA Dermatol. 2015;151(2):144–52. https://doi.org/10.1001/jamadermatol.2014.3059.
7. Guttman-Yassky E, Krueger JG, Lebwohl MG. Systemic immune mechanisms in atopic dermatitis and psoriasis with implications for treatment. Exp Dermatol. 2018;27(4):409–17. https://doi.org/10.1111/exd.13336.
8. Ungar B, Pavel AB, Robson PM, Kaufman A, Pruzan A, Brunner P, Kaushik S, Krueger JG, Lebwohl MG, Mani V, Fayad ZA, Guttman-Yassky E. A Preliminary $^{18}$F-FDG-PET/MRI Study Shows Increased Vascular Inflammation in Moderate-to-Severe Atopic Dermatitis. J Allergy Clin Immunol Pract. 2020;8(10):3500–6. https://doi.org/10.1016/j.jaip.2020.07.018.
9. Groenendyk JW, Shukla P, Dey AK, Elnabawi YA, Aksentijevich M, Choi H, Genovese LD, Harrington CL, Natarajan B, Goyal A, Reddy AS, Rodante J, Kabbany MT, Sadek A, Al Najafi M, Playford MP, Joshi AA, Ahlman MA, Gelfand JM, Bluemke DA, Mehta NN. Association of aortic vascular uptake of $^{18}$FDG by PET/CT and aortic wall thickness by MRI in psoriasis: a prospective observational study. Eur J Nucl Med Mol Imaging. 2019;46(12):2488–95. https://doi.org/10.1007/s00259-019-04454-w.
10. Yousuf O, Mohanty BD, Martin SS, Joshi PH, Blaha MJ, Nasir K, Blumenthal RS, Budoff MJ. High-sensitivity C-reactive protein and cardiovascular disease: a resolute belief or an elusive link? J Am Coll Cardiol. 2013;62(5):397–408. https://doi.org/10.1016/j.jacc.2013.05.016.
11. Strober B, Teller C, Yamauchi P, Miller JL, Hooper M, Yang YC, Dann F. Effects of etanercept on C-reactive protein levels in psoriasis and psoriatic arthritis. Br J Dermatol. 2008;159(2):322–30. https://doi.org/10.1111/j.1365-2133.2008.08628.x.
12. Vekaria AS, Brunner PM, Aleisa AI, Bonomo L, Lebwohl MG, Israel A, Guttman-Yassky E. Moderate-to-severe atopic dermatitis patients show increases in serum C-reactive protein levels, correlating with skin disease activity. F1000Res. 2017;6:1712. https://doi.org/10.12688/f1000research.12422.2.
13. Villani AP, Pavel AB, Wu J, Fernandes M, Maari C, Saint-Cyr Proulx E, Jack C, Glickman J, Choi S, He H, Ungar B, Estrada Y, Kameyama N, Zhang N, Gonzales J, Tardif JC, Krueger JG, Bissonnette R, Guttman-Yassky E. Vascular inflammation in moderate-to-severe atopic dermatitis is associated with enhanced Th2 response. Allergy. 2021;76(10):3107–21. https://doi.org/10.1111/all.14859.
14. Kim JD, Lee SH, Seo EH, Woo SY, Kim SH, Chung SM, Kim HJ. Role of Th1 and Th17 cells in the development and complexity of coronary artery disease: comparison analysis by the methods of flow cytometry and SYNTAX score. Coron Artery Dis. 2015;26(7):604–11. https://doi.org/10.1097/MCA.0000000000000289.
15. Taleb S. Inflammation in atherosclerosis. Arch Cardiovasc Dis. 2016;109(12):708–15. https://doi.org/10.1016/j.acvd.2016.04.002.
16. Hjuler KF, Böttcher M, Vestergaard C, Deleuran M, Raaby L, Bøtker HE, Iversen L, Kragballe K. Increased prevalence of coronary artery disease in severe psoriasis and severe atopic dermatitis. Am J Med. 2015;128(12):1325–34.e2. https://doi.org/10.1016/j.amjmed.2015.05.041.
17. Yamanaka KI, Mizutani H. The role of cytokines/chemokines in the pathogenesis of atopic dermatitis. Curr Probl Dermatol. 2011;41:80–92. https://doi.org/10.1159/000323299.
18. França CN, Izar MC, Amaral JB, Tegani DM, Fonseca FA. Microparticles as potential biomarkers of cardiovascular disease. Arq Bras Cardiol. 2015;104(2):169–74. https://doi.org/10.5935/abc.20140210.
19. Santilli F, Marchisio M, Lanuti P, Boccatonda A, Miscia S, Davì G. Microparticles as new markers of cardiovascular risk in diabetes and beyond. Thromb Haemost. 2016;116(2):220–34. https://doi.org/10.1160/TH16-03-0176.
20. Pelletier F, Garnache-Ottou F, Angelot F, Biichlé S, Vidal C, Humbert P, Saas P, Seillès E, Aubin F. Increased levels of circulating endothelial-derived microparticles and small-size platelet-derived microparticles in psoriasis. J Invest Dermatol. 2011;131(7):1573–6. https://doi.org/10.1038/jid.2011.57.

21. Pavel AB, Zhou L, Diaz A, Ungar B, Dan J, He H, Estrada YD, Xu H, Fernandes M, Renert-Yuval Y, Krueger JG, Guttman-Yassky E. The proteomic skin profile of moderate-to-severe atopic dermatitis patients shows an inflammatory signature. J Am Acad Dermatol. 2020;82(3):690–9. https://doi.org/10.1016/j.jaad.2019.10.039.
22. Furuhashi M. Fatty acid-binding protein 4 in cardiovascular and metabolic diseases. J Atheroscler Thromb. 2019;26(3):216–32. https://doi.org/10.5551/jat.48710.
23. Kjolby M, Nielsen MS, Petersen CM. Sortilin, encoded by the cardiovascular risk gene SORT1, and its suggested functions in cardiovascular disease. Curr Atheroscler Rep. 2015;17(4):496. https://doi.org/10.1007/s11883-015-0496-7.
24. Lee HJ, Hong YJ, Kim M. Angiogenesis in chronic inflammatory skin disorders. Int J Mol Sci. 2021;22(21):12035. https://doi.org/10.3390/ijms222112035.
25. Samochocki Z, Bogaczewicz J, Sysa-Jędrzejowska A, McCauliffe DP, Kontny E, Wozniacka A. Expression of vascular endothelial growth factor and other cytokines in atopic dermatitis, and correlation with clinical features. Int J Dermatol. 2016;55(3):e141–6. https://doi.org/10.1111/ijd.13132.
26. Zhang Y, Matsuo H, Morita E. Increased production of vascular endothelial growth factor in the lesions of atopic dermatitis. Arch Dermatol Res. 2006;297(9):425–9. https://doi.org/10.1007/s00403-006-0641-9.
27. Chang WL, Hsu MH, Lin CL, Chan PC, Chang KS, Lee CH, Hsu CY, Tsai MT, Yeh CH, Sung FC. Increased risk of stroke in contact dermatitis patients: a nationwide population-based retrospective cohort study. Medicine (Baltimore). 2017;96(10):e5650. https://doi.org/10.1097/MD.0000000000005650.
28. Tamagawa-Mineoka R, Katoh N, Ueda E, Masuda K, Kishimoto S. Elevated platelet activation in patients with atopic dermatitis and psoriasis: increased plasma levels of beta-thromboglobulin and platelet factor 4. Allergol Int. 2008;57(4):391–6. https://doi.org/10.2332/allergolint.O-08-537.
29. Nastałek M, Wojas-Pelc A, Undas A. Plasma fibrin clot properties in atopic dermatitis: links between thrombosis and atopy. J Thromb Thrombolysis. 2010;30(2):121–6. https://doi.org/10.1007/s11239-010-0478-0.
30. Oyoshi MK, He R, Kumar L, Yoon J, Geha RS. Cellular and molecular mechanisms in atopic dermatitis. Adv Immunol. 2009;102:135–226. https://doi.org/10.1016/S0065-2776(09)01203-6.

# Chapter 4
# AD and Psychodermatology/Quality of Life

**Marwa Hakimi, Kareem Elhage, Riley Spencer, Joy Jin, and Tina Bhutani**

**Case Title** A 24-year-old nursing student presents with an atopic dermatitis flare.

## Case

A 24-year-old nursing student with a history of mild atopic dermatitis presents to your dermatology office. She recently started clinical rotations in the hospital, which she reports is stressful. She reports feeling so itchy at night that she is unable to sleep. Physical exam reveals large erythematous lichenified plaques and multiple scattered excoriations on her hands, neck, antecubital fossa and behind her knees. The patient asks about how stress affects her atopic dermatitis. How do you respond?

## Board Review Question

A 16-year-old patient with atopic dermatitis reports that her classmates bully her because of the appearance of her skin. She feels embarrassed and hides her skin with long sleeve shirts and pants. What is the best next step?

A. Prescribe stronger topicals
B. Refer the patient to phototherapy

M. Hakimi (✉) · K. Elhage · R. Spencer · T. Bhutani
Department of Dermatology, University of California at San Francisco, San Francisco, CA, USA
e-mail: marwa.hakimi@ucsf.edu; kareem.elhage@med.wayne.edu; Riley.Spencer@ucsf.edu; Tina.Bhutani@ucsf.edu

J. Jin
Department of Dermatology, University of California at San Francisco, San Francisco, CA, USA

School of Medicine, University of California at San Francisco, San Francisco, CA, USA
e-mail: Joy.Jin@ucsf.edu



N. Brownstone et al. (eds.), *Clinical Cases in Atopic Dermatitis*, Clinical Cases in Dermatology, https://doi.org/10.1007/978-3-031-52147-8_4

C. Prescribe a JAK inhibitor
D. Screen for suicidality and make a mental health referral when necessary
E. Prescribe a biologic agent

## Main Text

There is a large burden of disease from atopic dermatitis on the lives of both patients and their families. The relationship between stress, mental health symptoms, and quality of life will be discussed in this chapter (Fig. 4.1).

### *Quality of Life*

The disease burden of atopic dermatitis (AD) can have a profound impact on quality of life. More than half of adults with AD reported that their skin condition limits their lifestyle [1]. Quality of life refers to an individual's overall sense of well-being and satisfaction with life, taking into account factors such as health, relationships, financial stability, and personal fulfillment. Health is a crucial component of quality of life as it affects an individual's ability to engage in daily activities, work, and overall function. Signs and symptoms related to uncontrolled AD such as pruritus, erythema, and sleep disturbance can be physically, socially, and emotionally debilitating, negatively affecting quality of life. The cycle of intense pruritus leading to scratching and further skin damage and inflammation can cause patients to experience pain, discomfort, and sleep disturbance. Furthermore, scratching can lead to skin infections that further exacerbate AD and require treatment. The demands of treatment and financial strain due to the high cost often also contribute to quality-of-life impairment. Given the variable intensity and frequency of AD, it requires

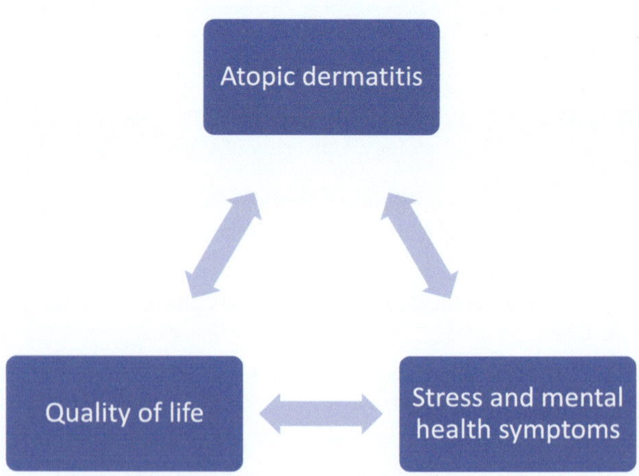


**Fig. 4.1** The connection between stress, mental health symptoms, and quality of life

regular healthcare visits and medications, which can be expensive and time-consuming. In severe cases, AD can affect a patient's ability to carry out daily activities interfering with work or school. In the United States, 43.3% of adults have reported that their AD impacts their activities [1]. Atopic dermatitis can have a significant emotional impact particularly on children and adolescents. The visible nature of AD can lead to embarrassment, shame, and feelings of self-consciousness generating a negative body image. Children with AD may avoid participating in social events to prevent others from seeing their condition. Conversely, AD patients may face discrimination and be excluded based on the visible nature of their disease leading to further social isolation. Adolescents and adults may experience difficulty forming relationships.

Quality-of-life measurements are an essential aspect of monitoring disease and treatment efficacy. The most frequently used are Children's Dermatology Life Quality Index (CDLQI), Dermatitis Family Index (DFI), Dermatology Life Quality Index (DLQI), and Infant Dermatitis Quality of Life Index (IDQoL) [2]. However, even if these are not available, healthcare providers can listen and ask questions to get a better understanding of how life with AD has been for their patients. In a population-based, cross-sectional study, adults with AD had significantly higher Dermatology Quality of Life Index scores and lower SF-12 mental health subscores [1]. These outcomes are associated with AD severity. A larger percentage of adults with AD reported being somewhat or very dissatisfied with life and having fair or poor health compared to those without AD [1]. The SF-12, a generic quality-of-life tool, mental health scores for moderate to severe AD were lower than other chronic health conditions like heart disease and diabetes, supporting the heavy burden that AD places on patients [1].

## *Stress*

Stress can be a trigger for atopic dermatitis flares, as it can disrupt and inhibit repair of the skin's barrier function leading to increased inflammation and induce the "itch-scratch cycle," worsening symptoms of atopic dermatitis. The constant pruritus and discomfort can make patients feel irritable and frustrated. A key pathway, the hypothalamic-pituitary-adrenal axis, is disturbed in atopic dermatitis affecting nerves, the immune system, and keratinocytes. Stress is a major contributor to aggravation of itch. Stress can lead to the production of cytokines and histamines, which also can result in increased itch. Itch then causes patients to scratch or rub the skin, which can lead to bleeding, infections, and scarring, amplifying the disease burden. This atopic dermatitis flare can then feedback and increase stress levels. Emotions such as frustration or embarrassment about the appearance of atopic dermatitis can increase stress levels and make symptoms worse. It is important for patients to identify and manage stress triggers to help improve atopic dermatitis symptoms and quality of life. Stress reduction techniques like cognitive behavioral therapy and habit reversal training can be helpful and are being studied in clinical trials. Massage therapy, acupuncture, and mindfulness-based stress reduction can reduce stress in AD patients as well [2]. For patients who may not be able to participate in formal stress relief training, instructions for how to perform simple actions such as alternate nasal breathing or progressive muscle relaxation can be helpful to reduce stress levels with regular use and practice.

## *Mental Health*

The connections between mental health issues and atopic dermatitis are an important, complex, and often unseen part of the disease burden. Adults with AD have up to a three-fold higher risk for anxiety or depression [3]. This could be due to the impact AD has on quality of life and the resulting social and emotional stress. Depression can result from social isolation and reduced participation in social activities that stems from the stigma of a visible chronic disease. Furthermore, sleep loss can influence practically all aspects of well-being including emotional state, mood, and the ability to concentrate. Sleep disturbance occurs in 67% of children and about one-third of adults with AD [4, 5]. Children with AD are up to six times more likely to have anxiety or depression than children without AD [6]. Furthermore, children with AD are more likely to be diagnosed with attention deficit hyperactivity disorder (ADHD) and other conduct disorders [7]. Assessing mental health in infants and young children is more difficult. Gaining better disease control may improve mental health in AD patients. Support groups and counseling services can also provide valuable resources for patients struggling with the psychological impact of AD. Dermatologists should have a low threshold to discuss a patient's mental health with their primary care physicians or refer to mental health providers.

## *Suicidality*

Suicidality describes suicidal ideation and the risk of attempting or completing suicide. Suicidal ideation refers to wishes, contemplations, and preoccupations with suicide and death or planning for suicide, while suicidal behavior includes attempting suicide or engaging in self-harming behaviors that may lead to suicide. Among adolescents, suicide is a leading cause of death with rates increasing in recent years [8]. Risk factors for suicidality include a history of suicide attempts, a family history of suicide, substance abuse, a recent loss or trauma, and chronic illness. Those suffering from AD are more likely to experience suicidal ideation (44% higher likelihood) and attempt suicide (36% higher likelihood) than those without AD [9]. Compared to healthy controls, female pediatric patients with AD have an increased risk of suicidal ideation and suicide attempts [10]. Although individuals with severe AD had higher suicidal ideation than individuals with mild AD, there was no difference when comparing incidence rates of completed suicides [11, 12]. It is critical that dermatology providers are aware of this increased risk in AD patients and appropriately screen, monitor, and refer to mental health providers. The National Suicide Prevention Lifeline in the United States, which can be accessed at 988, provides confidential support and resources.

## *Caregivers*

Quality-of-life impairment may also extend to caregivers, family members, and partners of those suffering from atopic dermatitis. There is an increase in caregiving responsibility because atopic dermatitis is a chronic condition that requires ongoing management. Caregivers may experience emotional stress seeing their loved one's struggle with the physical discomfort and embarrassment of atopic dermatitis and can even feel guilty if they are unable to provide relief. Caregivers' role may include helping to manage symptoms, applying topicals, coordinating appointments, care decision-making, helping to avoid triggers, emotional/mental support, and bearing the financial burden of paying for medication and healthcare visits, which can lead to financial strain and stress. Caregivers may miss work or experience decreased work productivity [13]. Caregivers may neglect their own self-care as they prioritize the needs of the person suffering from atopic dermatitis. Prioritizing their responsibilities over their social life can lead to feelings of loneliness and isolation. This can lead to physical and emotional exhaustion putting the caregiver's health at risk. It is important for caregivers to seek support and resources to manage their caregiving responsibilities and also take care of their own well-being.

**Board Review Question Explanation**

A 16-year-old patient with severe atopic dermatitis reports that her classmates bully her because of the appearance of her skin. She tries to cover her skin as much as possible. What is the next best step?

A. Prescribe stronger topicals
B. Refer the patient to phototherapy
C. Prescribe a JAK inhibitor
D. Screen for suicidality and make a mental health referral when necessary (correct)
E. Prescribe a biologic agent

**Explanation**

Increasing severity of atopic dermatitis and female sex are associated with an increased risk for both depression and suicidality. It is important to screen and assess psychiatric comorbidities in this patient as the best next step. Effective treatments can help alleviate some of the emotional burden associated with atopic dermatitis and would be the next step after screening for suicidality in this patient.

**Key Takeaway Points**

- Patients with AD have severe impacts on quality of life.
- Stress is a trigger for AD flares likely by leading to impairment in skin barrier function.

- AD symptoms can lead to further stress, thus creating a vicious cycle if the disease is not controlled adequately.
- Atopic dermatitis is associated with psychiatric comorbidities such as anxiety and depression.
- Individuals with atopic dermatitis are at significantly increased risk of suicidal ideation and suicide attempts.
- It is important for dermatologists to screen for quality of life and mental health impact of AD to determine disease burden, to identify patients requiring step-up treatment of their skin disease, and to refer patients to get additional help if needed.

## References

1. Silverberg JI, Gelfand JM, Margolis DJ, et al. Patient burden and quality of life in atopic dermatitis in US adults: a population-based cross-sectional study. Ann Allergy Asthma Immunol. 2018;121(3):340–7. https://doi.org/10.1016/j.anai.2018.07.006.
2. Rehal B, Armstrong AW. Health outcome measures in atopic dermatitis: a systematic review of trends in disease severity and quality-of-life instruments 1985–2010. [published correction appears in PLoS One. 2011;6(6): 10.1371/annotation/6d5e99c5-bd8f-4cef-b77a-fbb795633da0. Armstrong, April [Corrected to Armstrong, April W].]. PLoS One. 2011;6(4):e17520. https://doi.org/10.1371/journal.pone.0017520.
3. Silverberg JI, Gelfand JM, Margolis DJ, et al. Symptoms and diagnosis of anxiety and depression in atopic dermatitis in U.S. adults. Br J Dermatol. 2019;181(3):554–65. https://doi.org/10.1111/bjd.17683.
4. Fishbein AB, Cheng BT, Tilley CC, et al. Sleep disturbance in school-aged children with atopic dermatitis: prevalence and severity in a cross-sectional sample. J Allergy Clin Immunol Pract. 2021;9(8):3120–3129.e3. https://doi.org/10.1016/j.jaip.2021.04.064.
5. Silverberg JI, Garg NK, Paller AS, Fishbein AB, Zee PC. Sleep disturbances in adults with eczema are associated with impaired overall health: a US population-based study. J Invest Dermatol. 2015;135(1):56–66. https://doi.org/10.1038/jid.2014.325.
6. Yaghmaie P, Koudelka CW, Simpson EL. Mental health comorbidity in patients with atopic dermatitis. J Allergy Clin Immunol. 2013;131(2):428–33. https://doi.org/10.1016/j.jaci.2012.10.041.
7. Strom MA, Fishbein AB, Paller AS, Silverberg JI. Association between atopic dermatitis and attention deficit hyperactivity disorder in U.S. children and adults. Br J Dermatol. 2016;175(5):920–9. https://doi.org/10.1111/bjd.14697.
8. Centers for Disease Control and Prevention. Suicide rising across the US. https://www.cdc.gov/vitalsigns/suicide/. 2018. Accessed 8 Jan 2023.
9. Sandhu JK, Wu KK, Bui TL, Armstrong AW. Association between atopic dermatitis and suicidality: a systematic review and meta-analysis. JAMA Dermatol. 2019;155(2):178–87. https://doi.org/10.1001/jamadermatol.2018.4566.
10. Noh HM, Cho JJ, Park YS, Kim JH. The relationship between suicidal behaviors and atopic dermatitis in Korean adolescents. J Health Psychol. 2016;21(10):2183–94. https://doi.org/10.1177/1359105315572453.
11. Kimata H. Prevalence of suicidal ideation in patients with atopic dermatitis. Suicide Life Threat Behav. 2006;36(1):120–4. https://doi.org/10.1521/suli.2006.36.1.120.

12. Thyssen JP, Hamann CR, Linneberg A, et al. Atopic dermatitis is associated with anxiety, depression, and suicidal ideation, but not with psychiatric hospitalization or suicide. Allergy. 2018;73(1):214–20. https://doi.org/10.1111/all.13231.
13. Yang EJ, Beck KM, Sekhon S, Bhutani T, Koo J. The impact of pediatric atopic dermatitis on families: a review. Pediatr Dermatol. 2019;36(1):66–71. https://doi.org/10.1111/pde.13727.

# Chapter 5
# AD, Environment, and Diet

**Mitchell Davis, Tina Bhutani, and Wilson Liao**

**Case Title** A 19-year-old male presents with a long history of atopic dermatitis that flares in wintertime.

**Case**

A 19-year-old male presents with moderate atopic dermatitis (AD) that has waxed and waned since childhood. Upon discussing potential triggers with the patient, he reports that his AD flares in wintertime with cold and dry weather and improves in the summer with warm and humid environments. He also tells you that he thinks certain foods trigger AD flares. He asks you about the role of diet and environment in AD. How do you respond?

**Board Review Question**

A 19-year-old male presents with moderate atopic dermatitis (AD) that has waxed and waned since childhood. Upon discussing potential triggers with the patient, he reports that his AD flares in wintertime with cold and dry weather and improves in the summer with warm and humid environments. The patient has tried and failed topical steroids and calcineurin inhibitors and is reluctant to try a systematic agent at this time. Which of the following options would be a good next step in therapy?

A. Phototherapy
B. Topical tacrolimus
C. Dupilumab
D. Tralokinumab
E. Topical triamcinolone

M. Davis (✉) · T. Bhutani · W. Liao
Department of Dermatology, University of California, San Francisco, San Francisco, CA, USA
e-mail: Mitchell.Davis@ucsf.edu; Tina.Bhutani@ucsf.edu; wilson.liao@ucsf.edu



N. Brownstone et al. (eds.), *Clinical Cases in Atopic Dermatitis*, Clinical Cases in Dermatology, https://doi.org/10.1007/978-3-031-52147-8_5

## Introduction

The relationships between the environment, diet, and AD are particularly complex. Patients suffering from AD often ask their clinicians if various foods and climates could be negatively affecting their condition. Here, we discuss how various environmental and dietary factors may or may not affect AD.

## Impact of Environment on AD

A variety of factors have been theorized to be associated with the exacerbation of AD. One factor that has been of particular concern in recent years is the effect of global climate change on AD. In particular, there is a growing concern on the effect of temperature on AD. Changes in humidity and atmospheric ultraviolet (UV) radiation levels are the consequence of increased greenhouse gas emissions and subsequent rising global temperatures [1]. Although there is a lack of data demonstrating the association between AD and global climate change, we know that cutaneous nerves, responsible for itch, are more active at higher temperatures [2]. Thus, the predominant symptom of AD may be exacerbated by changes in global climate.

### *Humidity*

AD prevalence has been shown to increase in the winter, likely due to a decrease in humidity and UV exposure [3]. It has been proposed that low humidity is a potential aggravating factor of AD as a result of the reduction of filaggrin expression and increased conversion of filaggrin to natural moisturizing factor (NMF) [4, 5].

### *UV Radiation*

UV radiation, both from natural and man-made sources, can have a beneficial effect on AD [6]. In one systematic review, 19 studies involving clinical UV radiation and AD were assessed. Narrowband ultraviolet B (nbUVB) and UVA1 demonstrated the greatest improvement of clinical signs and symptoms of AD [7]. Interestingly, children born in seasons of decreased UV radiation (autumn and winter) have an increased likelihood of AD compared to children born in the spring and summer.

UV radiation influences AD both directly and indirectly. UV radiation has an immunosuppressive effect on AD by potentiating the expression of skin barrier proteins, antimicrobial peptides, and lipids, as well as decreasing histamine release [6, 7]. Additionally, UV radiation promotes the conversion of a byproduct of filaggrin, trans-urocanic acid, into cis-urocanic acid, a compound with immunosuppressive properties [8].

There is also evidence to support UV radiation's ability to suppress the production of *Staphylococcus aureus* superantigen, which has been shown to trigger AD flares [9, 10]. Conversely, the reduction of UV radiation has been linked to the alteration of the skin microbiome and subsequent colonization of the skin with bacteria such as *S. aureus* [11–13].

In terms of systemic immunological effects, UV radiation has been shown to increase Treg cells and vitamin D production. This, in turn, leads to a downregulation of cell-mediated immune function [14, 15].

## Migration and Urbanization

The effect of migration and urbanization on AD has also been investigated. The International Study of Asthma and Allergies in Childhood (ISAAC) demonstrated worldwide variations in the prevalence of AD as it relates to socioeconomic status [16]. Countries designated as "low-income" have exhibited an increase in AD prevalence, while countries with higher-income settings did not [17].

## Air Pollution

Airborne pollution is suspected to negatively impact AD via multiple mechanisms [18]. Air pollutants such as traffic-related air pollution (TRAP), tobacco smoke, volatile organic compounds (VOC), and particulate matter (PM) disrupt the skin barrier by generating reactive oxygen species (ROS) and causing an epigenetic modification of the immune system. This epigenetic modification has been demonstrated in utero to cause a shift in the adaptive immunity toward a Th2 phenotype, subsequently instigating the development of a pro-inflammatory cytokine profile in infants [11].

In particular, exposure to PM is suggested to cause a decrease in structural protein (e.g., filaggrin) and has been shown to increase *S. aureus* colonization in mouse models [19–21]. Exposure to VOC has been shown to affect AD by causing transepidermal water loss (TEWL) via an unknown mechanism. [20, 21] Additionally, a significant positive association between TRAP and AD was reported in a German study that followed women in rural and urban areas [18, 22]. Interestingly, certain women carrying a minor allele single nucleotide polymorphism in the aryl hydrocarbon receptor (AhR) gene were more likely to develop AD symptoms from TRAP [22]. Thus, AhR signaling may be involved in TRAP-induced eczematous symptoms [ 22].

## *Water Hardness*

An association between water hardness and AD has been demonstrated in cohort and cross-sectional studies [23, 24]. In patients with filaggrin gene (FLG) mutations who are exposed to hard water, a 23.3% increase in TEWL has been demonstrated [25]. When the skin is exposed to hard water, sodium lauryl sulfate (SLS) is deposited into the epidermal layer. SLS is suspected to downregulate profilaggrin expression and increase protease activity [8, 26, 27]. One Japanese study demonstrated that out-in skin transparency (OIST), a measurement used to assess how readily substances move across the stratum corneum, differed between individuals exposed to hard water and individuals exposed to soft water [28]. Those who were exposed to hard water exhibited lower OIST, indicating impairment of the skin tissue's ability to retain water. Additionally, subjective symptoms were evaluated using the visual analog scale (VAS). Statistically significant differences in pruritus and satisfaction with therapy were demonstrated [ 28].

## *Genetic Variation and Environment*

AD is characterized by multiple phenotypes and subtypes that differ based on factors such as ethnicity, disease chronicity, age, and underlying molecular mechanisms [29]. Ideally, clinicians would be able to practice precision medicine and allow individual patients to receive tailored treatment according to their unique AD phenotype. For example, AD patients may significantly differ in terms of IgE levels and filaggrin mutation (FLG) status [29].

The integrity of a patient's skin barrier may be compromised by reduced expression of structural skin proteins such as E-cadherin, cytokeratin, and filaggrin. Thus, the inheritance of loss-of-function mutations (e.g., FLG) is associated with AD, particularly disease diagnosed at a young age [11, 30]. This highlights the link between genetic predisposition and environmental factors in causing allergic sensitization. A defective skin barrier enables permeability to allergens and dysbiotic bacteria and instigates a Th2-polarized immune response [11]. A sensitized individual with compromised skin barrier function is inevitably exposed to food and aeroallergens, which cross the epidermis and perpetuate inflammation [11]. In a study published in 2015, adult individuals with AD and verified IgE sensitization to grass allergen were exposed to two consecutive days of pollen grains or clean air. Those who were exposed to the pollen grains demonstrated an increase in the scoring of AD (SCORAD) compared to the control arm of the study. The active arm also demonstrated increases in levels of CCL17, CCL22, and IL-4 [31].

## *Skin Microbiome*

Healthy skin microbiome is diverse and typically constituted by four dominant phyla: *Bacteroidetes*, *Actinobacteria*, *Proteobacteria*, and *Firmicutes* [32]. The skin in AD demonstrates reduced commensal diversity and an increase in *staphylococcal* species (e.g., *S. aureus*). [33] Factors such as alterations in pH, humidity, temperature, and exposure to antibiotics can alter the composition of bacterial populations on the skin [34]. *S. aureus*, in particular, may induce a Th2-type lymphocyte response and produce superantigens and toxins that damage the epidermal layer of the skin [35, 36]. The creation of antimicrobial peptides by commensal bacteria is reduced and compromises the skin further [ 37].

## Diet

A significant percentage of patients inquire about the relationship between food and AD [38]. The prevalence of food allergies (FA) and AD may be as high as 50.7% [39]. One systematic review demonstrated a link between increasing AD severity and chronicity with food sensitization and allergy [40]. In this review, AD typically preceded the findings of food sensitization and allergy [40]. An epidemiological study in Canada demonstrated that infants with AD who were sensitized to more than one airborne or food allergen by the age of 3 had a higher likelihood of developing allergic comorbidities when compared to infants who were monosensitized or non-sensitized [41]. A compromised skin barrier in AD may result in transcutaneous sensitization to allergens from food [10].

Although diet has long been a target of investigation in the field of atopic diseases, the connection remains incompletely understood. This is likely complicated by the expansive variety of food possibilities and the number of potential skin reactions to food. This complexity may inhibit the typical patient's understanding of the relationship of food to their AD symptoms. For example, food may be involved in conditions such as celiac disease, anaphylaxis, irritant contact dermatitis, and food intolerance [42]. Patients often mistakenly refer to all such reactions as food allergies. True food allergies are much less prevalent than patients assume. In one study where 20% of the population reported a food intolerance, 1% had a true IgE-mediated allergy upon testing [43]. Unfortunately, there are issues with testing for true IgE-mediated food allergies. Skin prick testing and serum-specific IgE (sIgE) are commonly utilized. However, SPT has a positive predictive value below 50%, and AD is not an IgE-mediated allergic condition [10]. The current gold standard for food allergies is the double-blind, placebo-controlled food challenge, a cumbersome procedure requiring clinical supervision [10].

Providers and patients frequently trial elimination diets and engage in excessive testing, often overlooking effective treatments for AD [10]. Thus, patients may significantly alter their diet and, to a degree, lifestyle, all while receiving no appreciable benefit [44]. In fact, there is evidence that elimination diets may lead to new IgE-mediated FAs to previously tolerated foods [45, 46]. In addition, elimination diets may cause nutritional deficiencies and unnecessary stress, particularly in children [10]. In 2012, a Joint Task Force (JTF) was created that included experts in the fields of asthma, allergy, and immunology. One of their missions was to develop recommendations for AD diagnosis and treatment [47]. In 2014, the American Academy of Dermatology (AAD) also created atopic dermatitis management guidelines. Both sets of guidelines included recommendations for the avoidance of elimination diets based on allergy testing [10, 47, 48].

One study investigated the relationship between food allergies and AD by conducting food challenge tests in patients with and without a history of AD. In this study, when children reported AD flare-ups as the singular symptom of food allergy, there was no statistically significant difference in reaction to food challenges between the AD arm and the placebo arm [49]. However, in that same study, children with a history of AD were more likely to be sensitized to foods, even though that sensitization did not manifest with symptoms [49].

## Gut Microbiome

Additionally, an alteration in gut microbiome diversity is hypothesized to be associated with AD because of its influence on systemic immunity [50, 51]. A diverse gut microbiome contributes to the maturation of Th1 and Treg pathways while suppressing aberrancies in the Th2 response [50, 51]. One experiment demonstrated that reduced TGF-beta signaling results in the reprogramming of Treg cells into Th2 cells via IL-4 signaling and expanded innate lymphoid cell 2 (ILC2) populations [52]. Supplementing with *Lactobacillus* strains in the diet appears to reverse these findings [5]. Unfortunately, the general use of pre- and probiotics has not been shown to have a significant effect on AD. One systematic review found that prebiotics did not cause a significant degree of risk reduction in cases of AD [53].

## Diet and Supplement Recommendations

Multiple studies have investigated the potential role of food, medications, and supplementation in improving and worsening AD symptoms [53–56]. In an international epidemiological study (ISAAC Phase One), a diet composed of a high amount of trans-fatty acids was associated with increased AD prevalence [54]. Exposure to antibiotics early in life and maternal exposure to antibiotics during late pregnancy are associated with higher rates of AD. [56, 57]

Multiple supplements and foods have been studied and shown potential benefits in the management of AD. In one particular open study in Japan, oolong tea, when combined with standard AD treatment (e.g., topical corticosteroids), was shown to have a beneficial effect in terms of visual assessment of disease extent and intensity of pruritus [58]. Similarly, in vitro and in vivo studies involving L-histidine have also shown a potential role for supplementation. [59] This enantiomer of the amino acid histidine is theorized to help in the management of AD by increasing filaggrin formation and, subsequently, skin barrier function [59]. Hempseed oil has also been demonstrated to decrease TEWL and potentially AD disease severity [60, 61]. Administration of this oil resulted in an increase in plasma levels of fatty acids, one of which, linoleic acid, is metabolically converted to a ceramide [60]. Also, a diet including unpasteurized milk has been associated with decreased AD prevalence [55]. Lastly, supplementation with vitamin E, vitamin D, or both has resulted in improvements in AD symptoms in multiple studies [61–65]. However, with the exception of possibly vitamin supplementation with vitamins D and E, the supplement studies demonstrating potential benefits do not demonstrate sufficient evidence for broad recommendation in the management of AD.

**Board Review Question Explanation**

A 19-year-old male presents with moderate atopic dermatitis (AD) that has waxed and waned since childhood. Upon discussing potential triggers with the patient, he reports that his AD flares in wintertime with cold and dry weather and improves in the summer with warm and humid environments. The patient has tried and failed topical steroids and calcineurin inhibitors and is reluctant to try a systematic agent at this time. Which of the following options would be a good next step in therapy?

A. Phototherapy (correct)
B. Topical tacrolimus
C. Dupilumab
D. Tralokinumab
E. Topical triamcinolone

**Explanation**

The exacerbation of this patient's symptoms in wintertime and the reported improvement of symptoms in summertime likely indicate that the patient would be a good candidate for phototherapy treatment. Narrowband and broadband UVB have demonstrated efficacy in the management of AD. The patient reported failing topical steroids and calcineurin inhibitors, so topical triamcinolone or tacrolimus would not be good options. At this time, the patient is not willing to try a systemic agent such as dupilumab or tralokinumab.

**Key Takeaway Points**

- An increasing body evidence is revealing complex relationships between environmental exposures and AD.
- Skin barrier disruption and dysregulation of the immune system appear to be integral components in the interaction between environmental factors and AD.

- Exposure to UV radiation (environmental or clinical) has been shown to improve symptoms of AD.
- Although diet is connected to atopic dermatitis, the intricate relationship is often difficult to distinguish and navigate.
- Elimination diets or dietary exclusion are often unnecessary and can cause potential harm to patients.
- Clinicians should not allow the potential interaction of food with a patient's AD to distract them from implementing standard, effective AD treatments.
- The avoidance of certain foods and the initiation of oral supplementation may be useful in the prevention and management of concomitant atopic dermatitis and food allergies.

## References


1. Nguyen GH, Andersen LK, Davis MDP. Climate change and atopic dermatitis: is there a link? Int J Dermatol. 2019;58(3):279–82. https://doi.org/10.1111/ijd.14016.
2. James WD, Elston DM, Treat JR, Rosenbach MA. Andrews' diseases of the skin: clinical dermatology. Elsevier Health Sciences; 2019.
3. Hancox JG, Sheridan SC, Feldman SR, Fleischer AB. Seasonal variation of dermatologic disease in the USA: a study of office visits from 1990 to 1998. Int J Dermatol. 2004;43(1):6–11. https://doi.org/10.1111/j.1365-4632.2004.01828.x.
4. Cau L, Pendaries V, Lhuillier E, et al. Lowering relative humidity level increases epidermal protein deimination and drives human filaggrin breakdown. J Dermatol Sci. 2017;86(2):106–13. https://doi.org/10.1016/j.jdermsci.2017.02.280.
5. Lee MJ, Kang MJ, Lee SY, et al. Perturbations of gut microbiome genes in infants with atopic dermatitis according to feeding type. J Allergy Clin Immunol. 2018;141(4):1310–9. https://doi.org/10.1016/j.jaci.2017.11.045.
6. Pearse AD, Gaskell SA, Marks R. Epidermal changes in human skin following irradiation with either UVB or UVA. J Invest Dermatol. 1987;88(1):83–7. https://doi.org/10.1111/1523-1747.ep12465094.
7. Hong SP, Kim MJ, Jung MY, et al. Biopositive effects of low-dose UVB on epidermis: coordinate upregulation of antimicrobial peptides and permeability barrier reinforcement. J Invest Dermatol. 2008;128(12):2880–7. https://doi.org/10.1038/jid.2008.169.
8. Flohr C, Mann J. New insights into the epidemiology of childhood atopic dermatitis. Allergy. 2014;69(1):3–16. https://doi.org/10.1111/all.12270.
9. Byremo G, Rød G, Carlsen KH. Effect of climatic change in children with atopic eczema. Allergy. 2006;61(12):1403–10. https://doi.org/10.1111/j.1398-9995.2006.01209.x.
10. Rustad AM, Nickles MA, Bilimoria SN, Lio PA. The role of diet modification in atopic dermatitis: navigating the complexity. Am J Clin Dermatol. 2022;23(1):27–36. https://doi.org/10.1007/s40257-021-00647-y.
11. Stefanovic N, Irvine AD, Flohr C. The role of the environment and Exposome in atopic dermatitis. Curr Treat Options Allergy. 2021;8(3):222–41. https://doi.org/10.1007/s40521-021-00289-9.
12. Patra V, Byrne SN, Wolf P. The skin microbiome: is it affected by UV-induced immune suppression? Front Microbiol. 2016;7:1235. https://doi.org/10.3389/fmicb.2016.01235.
13. Tsakok T, Woolf R, Smith CH, Weidinger S, Flohr C. Atopic dermatitis: the skin barrier and beyond. Br J Dermatol. 2019;180(3):464–74. https://doi.org/10.1111/bjd.16934.

14. Hart PH, Gorman S, Finlay-Jones JJ. Modulation of the immune system by UV radiation: more than just the effects of vitamin D? Nat Rev Immunol. 2011;11(9):584–96. https://doi.org/10.1038/nri3045.
15. Ullrich SE, Byrne SN. The immunologic revolution: photoimmunology. J Invest Dermatol. 2012;132(3 Pt 2):896–905. https://doi.org/10.1038/jid.2011.405.
16. Asher MI, Stewart AW, Mallol J, et al. Which population level environmental factors are associated with asthma, rhinoconjunctivitis and eczema? Review of the ecological analyses of ISAAC phase one. Respir Res. 2010;11(1):8. https://doi.org/10.1186/1465-9921-11-8.
17. Odhiambo JA, Williams HC, Clayton TO, Robertson CF, Asher MI, ISAAC Phase Three Study Group. Global variations in prevalence of eczema symptoms in children from ISAAC phase three. J Allergy Clin Immunol. 2009;124(6):1251–1258.e23. https://doi.org/10.1016/j.jaci.2009.10.009.
18. Hendricks AJ, Eichenfield LF, Shi VY. The impact of airborne pollution on atopic dermatitis: a literature review. Br J Dermatol. 2020;183(1):16–23. https://doi.org/10.1111/bjd.18781.
19. Han RT, Kim HY, Ryu H, et al. Glyoxal-induced exacerbation of pruritus and dermatitis is associated with staphylococcus aureus colonization in the skin of a rat model of atopic dermatitis. J Dermatol Sci. 2018;90(3):276–83. https://doi.org/10.1016/j.jdermsci.2018.02.012.
20. Huss-Marp J, Eberlein-König B, Breuer K, et al. Influence of short-term exposure to airborne Der p 1 and volatile organic compounds on skin barrier function and dermal blood flow in patients with atopic eczema and healthy individuals. Clin Exp Allergy. 2006;36(3):338–45. https://doi.org/10.1111/j.1365-2222.2006.02448.x.
21. Pan TL, Wang PW, Aljuffali IA, Huang CT, Lee CW, Fang JY. The impact of urban particulate pollution on skin barrier function and the subsequent drug absorption. J Dermatol Sci. 2015;78(1):51–60. https://doi.org/10.1016/j.jdermsci.2015.01.011.
22. Schnass W, Hüls A, Vierkötter A, Krämer U, Krutmann J, Schikowski T. Traffic-related air pollution and eczema in the elderly: findings from the SALIA cohort. Int J Hyg Environ Health. 2018;221(6):861–7. https://doi.org/10.1016/j.ijheh.2018.06.002.
23. Engebretsen KA, Johansen JD, Kezic S, Linneberg A, Thyssen JP. The effect of environmental humidity and temperature on skin barrier function and dermatitis. J Eur Acad Dermatol Venereol. 2016;30(2):223–49. https://doi.org/10.1111/jdv.13301.
24. Perkin MR, Craven J, Logan K, et al. Association between domestic water hardness, chlorine, and atopic dermatitis risk in early life: a population-based cross-sectional study. J Allergy Clin Immunol. 2016;138(2):509–16. https://doi.org/10.1016/j.jaci.2016.03.031.
25. Jabbar-Lopez ZK, Craven J, Logan K, et al. Longitudinal analysis of the effect of water hardness on atopic eczema: evidence for gene-environment interaction. Br J Dermatol. 2020;183(2):285–93. https://doi.org/10.1111/bjd.18597.
26. Danby SG, Brown K, Wigley AM, et al. The effect of water hardness on surfactant deposition after washing and subsequent skin irritation in atopic dermatitis patients and healthy control subjects. J Invest Dermatol. 2018;138(1):68–77. https://doi.org/10.1016/j.jid.2017.08.037.
27. Törmä H, Lindberg M, Berne B. Skin barrier disruption by sodium lauryl sulfate-exposure alters the expressions of involucrin, transglutaminase 1, profilaggrin, and kallikreins during the repair phase in human skin in vivo. J Invest Dermatol. 2008;128(5):1212–9. https://doi.org/10.1038/sj.jid.5701170.
28. Togawa Y, Kambe N, Shimojo N, et al. Ultra-pure soft water improves skin barrier function in children with atopic dermatitis: a randomized, double-blind, placebo-controlled, crossover pilot study. J Dermatol Sci. 2014;76(3):269–71. https://doi.org/10.1016/j.jdermsci.2014.10.009.
29. Czarnowicki T, He H, Krueger JG, Guttman-Yassky E. Atopic dermatitis endotypes and implications for targeted therapeutics. J Allergy Clin Immunol. 2019;143(1):1–11. https://doi.org/10.1016/j.jaci.2018.10.032.
30. Smieszek SP, Welsh S, Xiao C, et al. Correlation of age-of-onset of atopic dermatitis with Filaggrin loss-of-function variant status. Sci Rep. 2020;10(1):2721. https://doi.org/10.1038/s41598-020-59627-7.

31. Werfel T, Heratizadeh A, Niebuhr M, et al. Exacerbation of atopic dermatitis on grass pollen exposure in an environmental challenge chamber. J Allergy Clin Immunol. 2015;136(1):96–103.e9. https://doi.org/10.1016/j.jaci.2015.04.015.
32. Powers CE, McShane DB, Gilligan PH, Burkhart CN, Morrell DS. Microbiome and pediatric atopic dermatitis. J Dermatol. 2015;42(12):1137–42. https://doi.org/10.1111/1346-8138.13072.
33. Kong HH, Oh J, Deming C, et al. Temporal shifts in the skin microbiome associated with disease flares and treatment in children with atopic dermatitis. Genome Res. 2012;22(5):850–9. https://doi.org/10.1101/gr.131029.111.
34. Nakatsuji T, Gallo RL. The role of the skin microbiome in atopic dermatitis. Ann Allergy Asthma Immunol. 2019;122(3):263–9. https://doi.org/10.1016/j.anai.2018.12.003.
35. Alexander H, Paller AS, Traidl-Hoffmann C, et al. The role of bacterial skin infections in atopic dermatitis: expert statement and review from the international eczema council skin infection group. Br J Dermatol. 2020;182(6):1331–42. https://doi.org/10.1111/bjd.18643.
36. Geoghegan JA, Irvine AD, Foster TJ. Staphylococcus aureus and atopic dermatitis: a complex and evolving relationship. Trends Microbiol. 2018;26(6):484–97. https://doi.org/10.1016/j.tim.2017.11.008.
37. Lai Y, Cogen AL, Radek KA, et al. Activation of TLR2 by a small molecule produced by Staphylococcus epidermidis increases antimicrobial defense against bacterial skin infections. J Invest Dermatol. 2010;130(9):2211–21. https://doi.org/10.1038/jid.2010.123.
38. Chan J, Ridd MJ. Beliefs and practices among adults with eczema and carers of children with eczema regarding the role of food allergy. Clin Exp Dermatol. 2019;44(7):e235–7. https://doi.org/10.1111/ced.13955.
39. Kwon J, Kim J, Cho S, Noh G, Lee SS. Characterization of food allergies in patients with atopic dermatitis. Nutr Res Pract. 2013;7(2):115–21. https://doi.org/10.4162/nrp.2013.7.2.115.
40. Tsakok T, Marrs T, Mohsin M, et al. Does atopic dermatitis cause food allergy? A systematic review. J Allergy Clin Immunol. 2016;137(4):1071–8. https://doi.org/10.1016/j.jaci.2015.10.049.
41. Dharma C, Lefebvre DL, Tran MM, et al. Patterns of allergic sensitization and atopic dermatitis from 1 to 3 years: effects on allergic diseases. Clin Exp Allergy. 2018;48(1):48–59. https://doi.org/10.1111/cea.13063.
42. Anvari S, Miller J, Yeh CY, Davis CM. IgE-mediated food allergy. Clin Rev Allergy Immunol. 2019;57(2):244–60. https://doi.org/10.1007/s12016-018-8710-3.
43. Young E, Stoneham MD, Petruckevitch A, Barton J, Rona R. A population study of food intolerance. Lancet. 1994;343(8906):1127–30. https://doi.org/10.1016/s0140-6736(94)90234-8.
44. Bath-Hextall F, Delamere FM, Williams HC. Dietary exclusions for improving established atopic eczema in adults and children: systematic review. Allergy. 2009;64(2):258–64. https://doi.org/10.1111/j.1398-9995.2008.01917.x.
45. Chang A, Robison R, Cai M, Singh AM. Natural history of food-triggered atopic dermatitis and development of immediate reactions in children. J Allergy Clin Immunol Pract. 2016;4(2):229–236.e1. https://doi.org/10.1016/j.jaip.2015.08.006.
46. Kraft MT, Prince BT. Atopic dermatitis is a barrier issue, not an allergy issue. Immunol Allergy Clin N Am. 2019;39(4):507–19. https://doi.org/10.1016/j.iac.2019.07.005.
47. Schneider L, Tilles S, Lio P, et al. Atopic dermatitis: a practice parameter update 2012. J Allergy Clin Immunol. 2013;131(2):295–9.e1–27. https://doi.org/10.1016/j.jaci.2012.12.672.
48. Sidbury R, Tom WL, Bergman JN, et al. Guidelines of care for the management of atopic dermatitis: section 4. Prevention of disease flares and use of adjunctive therapies and approaches. J Am Acad Dermatol. 2014;71(6):1218–33. https://doi.org/10.1016/j.jaad.2014.08.038.
49. Roerdink EM, Flokstra-de Blok BMJ, Blok JL, et al. Association of food allergy and atopic dermatitis exacerbations. Ann Allergy Asthma Immunol. 2016;116(4):334–8. https://doi.org/10.1016/j.anai.2016.01.022.
50. Abrahamsson TR, Jakobsson HE, Andersson AF, Björkstén B, Engstrand L, Jenmalm MC. Low diversity of the gut microbiota in infants with atopic eczema. J Allergy Clin Immunol. 2012;129(2):434–40., 400.e1–2. https://doi.org/10.1016/j.jaci.2011.10.025.

51. West CE, Jenmalm MC, Prescott SL. The gut microbiota and its role in the development of allergic disease: a wider perspective. Clin Exp Allergy. 2015;45(1):43–53. https://doi.org/10.1111/cea.12332.
52. Noval Rivas M, Burton OT, Oettgen HC, Chatila T. IL-4 production by group 2 innate lymphoid cells promotes food allergy by blocking regulatory T-cell function. J Allergy Clin Immunol. 2016;138(3):801–811.e9. https://doi.org/10.1016/j.jaci.2016.02.030.
53. Cuello-Garcia C, Fiocchi A, Pawankar R, et al. Prebiotics for the prevention of allergies: a systematic review and meta-analysis of randomized controlled trials. Clin Exp Allergy. 2017;47(11):1468–77. https://doi.org/10.1111/cea.13042.
54. Ellwood P, Asher MI, Björkstén B, Burr M, Pearce N, Robertson CF. Diet and asthma, allergic rhinoconjunctivitis and atopic eczema symptom prevalence: an ecological analysis of the international study of asthma and allergies in childhood (ISAAC) data. ISAAC phase one study group. Eur Respir J. 2001;17(3):436–43. https://doi.org/10.1183/09031936.01.17304360.
55. Perkin MR, Strachan DP. Which aspects of the farming lifestyle explain the inverse association with childhood allergy? J Allergy Clin Immunol. 2006;117(6):1374–81. https://doi.org/10.1016/j.jaci.2006.03.008.
56. Timm S, Schlünssen V, Olsen J, Ramlau-Hansen CH. Prenatal antibiotics and atopic dermatitis among 18-month-old children in the Danish National Birth Cohort. Clin Exp Allergy. 2017;47(7):929–36. https://doi.org/10.1111/cea.12916.
57. Pascal M, Perez-Gordo M, Caballero T, et al. Microbiome and allergic diseases. Front Immunol. 2018;9:1584. https://doi.org/10.3389/fimmu.2018.01584.
58. Uehara M, Sugiura H, Sakurai K. A trial of oolong tea in the management of recalcitrant atopic dermatitis. Arch Dermatol. 2001;137(1):42–3. https://doi.org/10.1001/archderm.137.1.42.
59. Tan SP, Brown SB, Griffiths CE, Weller RB, Gibbs NK. Feeding filaggrin: effects of l-histidine supplementation in atopic dermatitis. Clin Cosmet Investig Dermatol. 2017;10:403–11. https://doi.org/10.2147/CCID.S146760.
60. Callaway J, Schwab U, Harvima I, et al. Efficacy of dietary hempseed oil in patients with atopic dermatitis. J Dermatol Treat. 2005;16(2):87–94. https://doi.org/10.1080/09546630510035832.
61. Reynolds KA, Juhasz MLW, Mesinkovska NA. The role of oral vitamins and supplements in the management of atopic dermatitis: a systematic review. Int J Dermatol. 2019;58(12):1371–6. https://doi.org/10.1111/ijd.14404.
62. Amestejani M, Salehi BS, Vasigh M, et al. Vitamin D supplementation in the treatment of atopic dermatitis: a clinical trial study. J Drugs Dermatol. 2012;11(3):327–30.
63. Javanbakht MH, Keshavarz SA, Djalali M, et al. Randomized controlled trial using vitamins E and D supplementation in atopic dermatitis. J Dermatolog Treat. 2011;22(3):144–50. https://doi.org/10.3109/09546630903578566.
64. Sidbury R, Sullivan AF, Thadhani RI, Camargo CA. Randomized controlled trial of vitamin D supplementation for winter-related atopic dermatitis in Boston: a pilot study. Br J Dermatol. 2008;159(1):245–7. https://doi.org/10.1111/j.1365-2133.2008.08601.x.
65. Tsoureli-Nikita E, Hercogova J, Lotti T, Menchini G. Evaluation of dietary intake of vitamin E in the treatment of atopic dermatitis: a study of the clinical course and evaluation of the immunoglobulin E serum levels. Int J Dermatol. 2002;41(3):146–50. https://doi.org/10.1046/j.1365-4362.2002.01423.x.

# Chapter 6
# Treatment of AD with Non-pharmacological Interventions

**Madeleine Kilimnik and Elizabeth Jones**

**Case Title** A 6-year-old male with pruritic erythematous papules and plaques.

**Case**

A 6-year-old male presents to clinic with his parents. They have never been to the dermatologist before and explain that he has been scratching on and off for several years now, mostly in the flexural areas of his arms. On exam, you note erythematous papules and plaques on the flexor surfaces of his arms and popliteal fossa. The patient tells you he scratches them often. The parents bathe the patient daily before bed. He has no other medical conditions besides allergic rhinitis, for which he takes an antihistamine. The parents tell you they have not tried any treatments for his condition and are wondering about the next steps to take.

**Board Review Question**

A young female patient with a past medical history of allergic rhinitis and atopic dermatitis presents to clinic with significant pain and pruritus over significant portions of her body. Her parents tell you that they have not used regular moisturizing techniques or the topical agents prescribed during their last visit. The patient is reporting 10/10 pain, and the parents ask what they should do next.

M. Kilimnik
Sidney Kimmel Medical College, Philadelphia, PA, USA

E. Jones (✉)
Department of Dermatology, Thomas Jefferson University, Philadelphia, PA, USA
e-mail: Elizabeth.Jones@jefferson.edu



N. Brownstone et al. (eds.), *Clinical Cases in Atopic Dermatitis*, Clinical Cases in Dermatology, https://doi.org/10.1007/978-3-031-52147-8_6

A. Prescribe an oral steroid for them to use short term
B. Suggest wet wrap therapy to use in the acute setting and regular moisturizing thereafter
C. Wait for the flare to self-resolve
D. Tell them to only use a petrolatum moisturizer for the next few days
E. Tell them to only use a topical calcineurin inhibitor for the next few days

## Main Text

### *Moisturizing*

Consistent use of moisturizers is crucial in atopic dermatitis (AD) to decrease severity of disease. In AD, decreased filaggrin expression causes the skin to lose its barrier function and thus lose more water [1]. Losing a protective skin barrier allows allergens to penetrate the skin and cause inflammation and pruritus. Loss of barrier function also causes the skin to lose its protective function against infection [2]. Using a moisturizer helps to bring water to the skin surface, as well as create an occlusive barrier to prevent more water loss trans-epidermally. In doing so, the skin is able to protect the body from infection, as well as cause less disruption for the patient in regard to pain and pruritus [1, 2].

There are several different types of moisturizers to consider. Emollients contain long-chain saturated fatty acids, such as those in palm or coconut oil. These types of moisturizers are effective at increasing water retention in the stratum corneum by decreasing membrane permeability and increasing repair mechanisms. Humectants, such as 10% urea, contain emollient properties and also help bring additional moisture from the dermis into the stratum corneum. Humectants can cause extra moisture to evaporate from the skin as well, an issue addressed by simply adding an occlusive moisturizer on top of the humectant. Occlusives, like petroleum or lanolin, create a hydrophobic barrier and have the most significant impact on decreasing trans-epidermal water loss. Occlusive moisturizers are often thick and greasy and can be difficult for patients to tolerate for consistent use [1, 2].

Ceramides are an extremely beneficial ingredient in many moisturizers tailored toward AD patients [1]. Ceramides are crucial lipids responsible for barrier function and make up a significant proportion of the lipids in the stratum corneum. This helps both repair the stratum corneum and prevent water loss.

### *Bathing Practices*

Regarding bathing practices, it is important to educate the patient on the harmful effects of frequent wetting and drying of the skin, as well as the continuous use of soap. When bathing, if the patient is able to solely use soap on the apocrine areas of the skin, it would cause less moisture loss overall. The "soak and smear" technique refers to bathing, usually before bed time, and then not drying the skin immediately. The patient then would apply an ointment, such as a moisturizer or steroid-based formula, to the wet skin. This allows the skin to still contain the water from the bath while also allowing the AD to heal with the topical ointment or corticosteroid. Oftentimes, the corticosteroid application should be repeated in the morning [3].

A study showed that 28 patients with different dermatoses, such as AD, irritant dermatitis, psoriasis, nummular eczema, and xerotic eczema, were treated with the aforementioned "soak and smear" technique. Seventeen of the 28 patients showed a complete or nearly complete eradication of their dermatitis within several days to weeks of using the "soak and smear" technique [3]. A separate study of 55 children with AD showed no significant difference between applying topical steroids to pre-soaked vs. dry skin, so it is important to inform the patients of the significant results that use of topical steroids can have [4]. Another technique involves bathing in diluted bleach solution, which can help kill bacteria on the skin and prevent infection in AD patients.

## *Wet Wrap Therapy*

Wet wrap therapy describes the technique of leaving moist cloth or gauze on the skin for several hours or overnight to help with hydration during flares. In AD, the skin cannot retain moisture because the barrier function is compromised. Utilizing wet wrap therapy helps keep the skin moist. Proper use of wet wrap therapy includes first wetting cotton white clothing or gauze and wrapping it around the affected areas of the body. If the hands or feet are involved, cotton gloves or socks may be used. Once the wet layer is applied, a dry layer of gauze should be wrapped around, followed by dry clothing. If done at night, this can be dry pajamas. During the day, a track suit can be employed. Keeping the wet wrap on for several hours to overnight can help the skin regain some moisture and help with the pruritus and pain that usually accompany an AD flare (Table 6.1) [5].

Wet wrap therapy is traditionally used as a technique to provide relief during acute exacerbations of AD. However, a study analyzing the use of consistent wet

**Table 6.1** Steps for initiating wet wrap therapy during an AD flare

| | | |
|---|---|---|
| 1. | Wet dressing | Soak gauze or cotton clothing in warm water and wrap around the affected areas; for feet or hands, cotton gloves or socks can be used |
| 2. | Dry dressing | Place a dry wrapping over the wet gauze or clothing; vinyl gloves can be used on the hands and plastic wrap on the feet instead |
| 3. | Clothing | Wear dry pajamas or a track suit on top of this to prevent movement of the wrapping |
| 4. | Duration | Wear overnight or during the day for several hours for relief of AD symptoms |

wrap therapy for AD maintenance actually showed no significant difference compared to the placebo group in regard to overall clinical improvement and use of topical corticosteroids. The wet wrap therapy group had a greater incidence of secondary infection, and the therapy modality itself was difficult to implement on a regular basis [6].

## *Other Non-pharmacologic Treatments*

Other non-pharmacologic treatments for AD also exist beyond those mentioned previously in this section. There is limited or anecdotal evidence that the following treatments may work to help with AD: massage, acupuncture, yoga, tai chi, and mindfulness could be helpful, especially to prevent AD flares. There is an association between flares and stress levels, and it is thought that the aforementioned methods may help with stress reduction and, in doing so, reduce the extent of AD for patients. Beyond this, some patients use coconut or sunflower oil, which likely helps with hydration similarly to an occlusive moisturizer [7]. There are several vitamins and supplements that have been used by patients with AD, such as zinc, vitamin D, vitamin B12, fish oil, prebiotics and probiotics, turmeric, and CBD oil; of note, these only have limited data to support their use in AD [7, 8].

**Board Review Question Explanation**

A young female patient with a past medical history of allergic rhinitis and atopic dermatitis presents to clinic with significant pain and pruritus over significant portions of her body. Her parents tell you that they have not used regular moisturizing techniques or the topical agents prescribed during their last visit. The patient is reporting 10/10 pain, and the parents ask what they should do next.

A. Prescribe an oral steroid for them to use short term
B. Suggest wet wrap therapy to use in the acute setting and regular moisturizing thereafter (correct)
C. Wait for the flare to self-resolve
D. Tell them to only use a petrolatum moisturizer for the next few days
E. Tell them to only use a topical calcineurin inhibitor for the next few days

**Explanation**

Wet wrap therapy is traditionally used as a technique to provide relief during acute exacerbations of AD.

**Key Takeaway Points**

- The mainstay treatment of atopic dermatitis is regular and proactive use of moisturizers.
- Bathing techniques like the "soak and smear technique" can allow the skin to better retain moisture.

- Wet wrap therapy can provide significant relief to patients during atopic dermatitis flares.
- Other non-pharmacologic treatments like exercise techniques, oils, and vitamins have been reported to be beneficial in limited capacities.

## References


1. Purnamawati S, Indrastuti N, Danarti R, Saefudin T. The role of moisturizers in addressing various kinds of dermatitis: a review. Clin Med Res. 2017;15(3–4):75–87.
2. Giam YC, Hebert AA, Dizon MV, Van Bever H, Tiongco-Recto M, Kim KH, Soebono H, Munasir Z, Diana IA, Luk DC. A review on the role of moisturizers for atopic dermatitis. Asia Pac Allergy. 2016;6(2):120–8.
3. Gutman AB, Kligman AM, Sciacca J, James WD. Soak and smear: a standard technique revisited. Arch Dermatol. 2005;141(12):1556–9.
4. Kohn LL, et al. A randomized, controlled trial comparing topical steroid application to wet versus dry skin in children with atopic dermatitis. J Am Acad Dermatol. 2016;75:306–11.
5. National Eczema Association. Wet wrap therapy. (2022). https://nationaleczema.org/eczema/treatment/wet-wrap-therapy/. Accessed 13 Jan 2023.
6. Hindley D, Galloway G, Murray J, Gardener L. A randomised study of "wet wraps" versus conventional treatment for atopic eczema. Arch Dis Child. 2006;91(2):164–8.
7. National Eczema Association. Can natural treatments help manage your eczema? (2022. https://nationaleczema.org/eczema/treatment/complementary-and-alternative/. Accessed 13 Jan 2023.
8. Januchowski R. Evaluation of topical vitamin B(12) for the treatment of childhood eczema. J Altern Complement Med. 2009;15(4):387–9.

# Chapter 7
# Treatment of AD with Topical Therapy

**Kripa Ahuja and Peter Lio**

**Case Title** A 15-year-old female presents with an oozing, weeping rash and excoriations.

**Case**

It's Friday morning, and your first patient of the day is a teenager who presents with a 4-month history of a "red, itchy rash." The eruption is not well-defined, mildly edematous, and erythematous, with small erosions present. The rash is concentrated on the flexor surfaces, in particular the antecubital fossae and ventral wrists. The patient states that the rash gets worse in the winter. Upon asking the patient about her previous medical history, you learn she has a history of asthma and is "allergy prone." Based on her clinical presentation and history, the diagnosis at the top of your list is atopic dermatitis (AD). You have a medical student doing a dermatology rotation with you. He asks you the best treatment practices for AD. How do you respond to this medical student?

**Board Review Question**

Which of the following are possible side effects from topical corticosteroids?

A. Steroid-induced acne
B. Dermal atrophy
C. Chronic lichenification
D. Cushing's disease
E. A, C, and E
F. A, B, and D

K. Ahuja
Eastern Virginia Medical School, Norfolk, VA, USA

P. Lio (✉)
Department of Dermatology, Northwestern University, Chicago, IL, USA



N. Brownstone et al. (eds.), *Clinical Cases in Atopic Dermatitis*, Clinical Cases in Dermatology, https://doi.org/10.1007/978-3-031-52147-8_7

Atopic dermatitis (AD) is a chronic, pruritic, inflammatory disorder that often presents with comorbid allergic conditions. An interplay of dysregulated immune function, skin barrier, genetics, and environmental factors contributes to AD. Increased interleukin 4 (IL-4) and interleukin 13 (IL-13) drive the Th2 response. While inflammation certainly plays a key role in AD, there are other pathogenic factors involved as well. Skin barrier dysfunction is thought to be at the core of AD, if not as a primary problem, then invariably as a secondary one. Genetic defects in filaggrin, chronic irritants, psychological or physical stress, harsh climates, pollutants, diet, and a multitude of different components are implicated in skin barrier dysfunction leading to AD. Overall, abnormal immune responses and skin barrier dysfunction drive the pathogenesis of AD. Therefore, treatments are often aimed at these two aspects, with the goal being to reduce symptoms, prevent flares, and improve quality of life. While there are a variety of non-pharmacologic approaches for AD and while good education, avoidance of known triggers, and gentle skin care are important for all patients, we will discuss four key pharmacological agents used to treat AD topically: corticosteroids, crisaborole, calcineurin inhibitors, and Janus kinase (JAK) inhibitors.

Many guideline documents separate treatments by severity and typically place topical agents in the mild or moderate categories, reserving systemic agents for the severe category. However, assessing disease severity in AD is deceptively complex. While validated scales such as the Investigator's Global Assessment (IGA, more recently rebranded as the vIGA-AD) exist, they have a number of limitations including but not limited to:

- AD can change appearance within days and perhaps even in hours, making a "point estimation" of somewhat limited value.
- Many tools measure only clinically apparent signs and ignore symptoms and impact on quality of life.
- Some tools such as IGA do not account for body surface area involvement, which can have a dramatic effect on treatment selection.

Better tools exist but are beyond the scope of this chapter, and perhaps it is best noted that, regardless of severity, topical therapy is almost always warranted consideration, even when used as an adjunct to systemic therapies.

## Corticosteroids

The mechanism of action for corticosteroids is multifactorial, but they bind to a nuclear receptor to inhibit pro-inflammatory transcription factors, including nuclear factor kappa B (NFkB) and nuclear factor of activated T cells (NFAT). The inhibition of these transcription factors leads to a downstream effect of decreasing synthesis and release of prostaglandins, leukotrienes, and inflammatory cytokines via blockade of phospholipase A2. Additionally, functional changes occur in endothelial cells, granulocytes, T cells, mast cells, and Langerhans cells. At the epidermal level, the mitotic activity of epidermal cells and dermal fibroblasts is inhibited.

Another important mechanism of action for corticosteroids is their vasoconstrictive effect. The vasoconstrictive effect correlates with corticosteroids' anti-inflammatory efficacy. A hallmark of inflammation is vasodilation, either acute or chronic. When vessels are dilated, they are exposed to increased wall tension and stretch force. It is precisely this physical stretch of the blood vessel walls and endothelium that has experimentally been shown to result in increased production of pro-inflammatory cytokines: vascular endothelial growth factor (VEGF), tumor necrosis factor α (TNFα), monocyte chemoattractant protein (MCP-1), interleukin 6 (IL-6), and interleukin 8 (IL-8). Experimentally, increased wall tension can result in opening usually closed gaps in vessel walls. This opening then leads to fluid and inflammatory cells moving into the surrounding areas. Thus, when corticosteroids vasoconstrict vessels, there is a decrease in vessel diameter, resulting in decreased wall tension. The decreased wall tension leads to decreased synthesis of pro-inflammatory cytokines and decreased movement of fluid and inflammatory cells, thereby decreasing inflammation.

When steroids are applied to the skin, they are cutaneously absorbed and diffused to the dermal vasculature resulting in superficial vasoconstriction. In simple terms, vasoconstriction leads to decreased blood flow, and the skin "blanches." The vasoconstrictor assay, also known as the human skin blanching assay, was described by Mckenzie and Stoughton in 1962. This assay, often referred to as the "Stoughton scale," consists of applying a topical steroid to the volar arm with a subsequent observation of the level of vasoconstriction. There are four levels ranging from no vasoconstriction to strong vasoconstriction. The topical potency, bioavailability, and strength of penetration are all based on the vasoconstrictor assay. In fact, the Food and Drug Administration (FDA) uses this assay to assess the bioavailability and bioequivalence of different TCS.

When choosing a topical steroid, the patient's age, region of the body, and degree of skin inflammation should be considered. In particular, the face, genitals, and skin folds are at high risk for atrophy when treated with steroids. Historical treatment of AD has focused on topical steroid treatment of visible skin lesions: the more severe the lesion, the stronger the steroid. After the visible skin lesions disappeared, the topical steroid would be tapered down to be eventually stopped, replaced by emollients that stabilize the skin barrier. This approach to treatment of AD is referred to as "reactive therapy." There are various pros and cons of reactive therapy. Reactive therapy is generally effective at clearing flares of acute eczema and aims to minimize exposure to medications. However, a downfall of this approach is that recurrences after short-term improvement are common, and it lacks a strategy to address long-term control of flares. In milder disease, cessation of the steroid and possible recurrences can be managed by proper skin care and emollient use. However, for some patients, cessation of the steroid can result in an immediate and severe eczema flare, sometimes even worse than the baseline disease that was initially being treated. This is referred to as a "rebound flare" and can be disastrous for some patients leading to overreliance and overuse of topical steroids.

In such cases, the concept of "proactive therapy" emerges as an attractive alternative. Recent literature has focused on using topical steroids or non-steroidal agents as "proactive therapy," especially in more recalcitrant cases. Whereas reactive therapy focuses on the cessation of steroids when the skin begins to look clear to the naked eye, proactive therapy reminds us that the clinically "non-lesional" skin in AD is still abnormal due to various pathophysiological defects and often has underlying inflammation. Proactive therapy is similar to reactive therapy in that more powerful treatments—generally topical steroids—are used to clear the flare. However, it differs from reactive therapy in that a low-dose steroid (or, as will be discussed later, a non-steroidal agent) is applied intermittently for a longer term, along with emollients to maintain calm skin and help prevent a disease flare. This type of therapy can be described as "minimal therapy for minimal eczema." It will not be stopped after lesions visibly disappear but will be continued at a low frequency, usually twice a week.

Data from different trials using proactive therapy with TCS have shown a significant improvement in skin lesions, a significant reduction of flares, and an overall better quality of life for the patients. This type of therapy also empowers the patient, as the patient controls the disease and *prevents* flares, as opposed to simply treating the flares after they have already occurred.

Topical corticosteroids are not without side effects. Following daily application, atrophy of the skin along with telangiectasia and striae can occur as quickly as 2–3 weeks after starting therapy. However, the skin can recover relatively quickly after cessation of therapy. Systemic absorption can occur, particularly with the use of super-high-potency and high-potency corticosteroids, and can result in adrenal suppression, hyperglycemia, and growth abnormalities, especially if used in children.

Topical steroid withdrawal syndrome (TSWS) is a somewhat controversial phenomenon. TSWS is different than pharmacologic withdrawal of a steroid, which can lead to a "rebound" flare of the AD—it can persist and involve new areas with new morphologies sometimes for years after cessation of corticosteroids. TSWS occurs most often on the face, and it seems to affect females in a greater proportion than males. Clinicians should be aware of the presentation of topical steroid withdrawal syndrome and educate patients accordingly. While treatment for TSWS is not yet standardized, new studies are being conducted on TSWS. While this is still a somewhat controversial entity, it is worth being aware of for anyone who might prescribe TCS. It also underscores the importance for having non-steroidal options in our therapeutic armamentarium (Fig. 7.1).

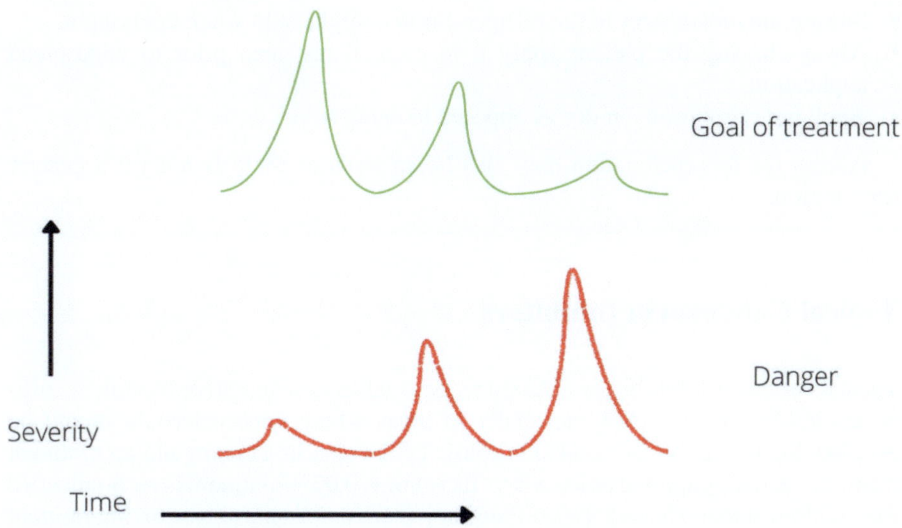


**Fig. 7.1** Goal of treatment of AD with topical steroids

## Crisaborole (PDE4)

Crisaborole is a topical phosphodiesterase (PDE4) inhibitor that is approved for treatment of mild to moderate AD in adults and children down to 3 months of age. Crisaborole uses boron-based chemistry to inhibit PDE4 in a reversible, competitive manner. When the PDE4 enzyme is inhibited, it negatively regulates cytokines including IL-4 and IL-13, which are implicated in the pathogenesis of AD. Crisaborole comes in a 2% ointment formulation.

In the United States, it is approved for the treatment of mild to moderate AD, and clinically the efficacy is perhaps closer to a low-potency corticosteroid. A 2021 comparative trial evaluated crisaborole against two topical calcineurin inhibitors: pimecrolimus 1% and tacrolimus 0.03%. The trial evaluated each drug's efficacy in treating mild to moderate AD via the Investigator's Static Global Assessment (ISGA). The trial found crisaborole to have higher odds of improving ISGA score compared to pimecrolimus 1% or tacrolimus 0.03% in patients over 2 years old with mild to moderate AD.

The most common side effects of crisaborole are application site reactions, including burning and stinging. While crisaborole is a novel, effective drug, the application site reactions are important to anticipate. To minimize application site pain, we have used some of the following practices with favorable results:

- Using a topical steroid a few days prior to starting treatment with crisaborole to "cool" the inflammation before applying it.
- Applying moisturizer before applying crisaborole.

- Storing the moisturizer in the refrigerator to cool the skin when applying it.
- Always having the patient apply it to a small test area prior to widespread application.
- Applying crisaborole on dry as opposed to damp skin.

Access for this medication may also be an issue as there is not yet a generic formulation.

## Topical Calcineurin Inhibitors

Topical calcineurin inhibitors (TCIs) can be used as an alternative to topical corticosteroids for treating AD, especially in areas where corticosteroids should be avoided, including the face and skin folds. TCIs come in a cream and an ointment formulation that is applied twice a day. Tacrolimus 0.03% ointment is recommended for children under 16 with twice daily application for short-term or intermittent long-term use, while the 0.1% ointment formulation is indicated for ages 16 and over. One percent pimecrolimus cream is approved for ages 2 years and up. Tacrolimus is indicated for moderate to severe AD, while pimecrolimus is for mild to moderate disease.

Topical calcineurin inhibitors work by inhibiting T-cell activation. Specifically, they bind cytosolic proteins such as cyclophilin and FK-binding proteins. When the drugs bind these cytosolic proteins, the drug-receptor complex specifically and competitively binds and inhibits calcineurin, a calcium- and calmodulin-dependent phosphatase. When calcineurin is inhibited, the translocation of the NF-AT transcription factors is inhibited. Therefore, the transcription of T-cell-activating interleukins (interleukin 2) and pro-inflammatory cytokines (tumor necrosis factor $\alpha$, interleukin 4, interleukin 3, granulocyte-macrophage colony-stimulating factor, and interferon-gamma) is inhibited.

Due to their mechanism of action, there is a possible concern that TCIs might lead to increased lymphoma and skin cancer rates. Fortunately, recent longitudinal studies have not found increased cancer rates in children using TCIs in AD. The APPLES study (A Prospective Pediatric Longitudinal Evaluation to Assess the Long-Term Safety of Tacrolimus Ointment for the Treatment of Atopic Dermatitis) is a landmark, international longitudinal study published in 2020 examining the incidence of cancer in nearly 8000 children treated with 0.03% or 0.1% tacrolimus ointment. The study found that neither tacrolimus treatment for AD nor AD itself increased the risk for malignancy.

Similar to the proactive therapy method mentioned with TCS, studies show that proactive therapy with 0.1% tacrolimus ointment has a statistically significant reduction in the flares of AD for adults and children. Studies also show that proactive therapy with 0.1% tacrolimus prolonged the time to flare in children. There are no studies to date directly comparing proactive therapy with TCI against TCS.

The main side effects of TCIs include reaction site pain, particularly burning. While studies have found TCIs to be comparable to TCS in treating AD, the reported side effect of application site burning is far greater in TCIs. Another notable side effect of topical calcineurin inhibitors seen in a certain percentage of patients is facial flushing with alcohol ingestion. The facial erythema may be due to tacrolimus-induced release of substance P or alcohol-induced vasodilation; however, the complete pathophysiology is not understood. Providers should be aware of this potentially socially stigmatizing effect and educate patients accordingly.

## Janus Kinase Inhibitors

The Janus kinases (JAK) are a group of molecules, including JAK1, JAK2, JAK3, and tyrosine kinase (TYK2), that are crucial for the activation of transcription of many critical pro-inflammatory cytokines that are involved in the pathogenesis of AD including interferon-$\gamma$ (IFN-$\gamma$), interleukin 4 (IL-4), interleukin 13 (IL-13), interleukin 31 (IL-31), interleukin 33 (IL-33), interleukin 23 (IL-23), interleukin 22 (IL-22), and interleukin 17 (IL-17). Various JAK inhibitors target different components of the JAK system. Topical ruxolitinib is a JAK1 and JAK2 inhibitor that produces rapid and sustained antipruritic and anti-inflammatory effects. Topical ruxolitinib appears to be comparable to the mid-potency TCS triamcinolone in efficacy, and a further advantage of this drug over TCS is the lack of class-associated side effects such as skin atrophy and ocular risks. The most common adverse effect of topical JAK inhibitors was application site reaction. The JAK inhibitors are a new class of drugs that lack long-term studies in treating AD.

## Therapeutic Education

In addition to these primary treatment modalities, patient education regarding AD is vital.

Clinicians should educate patients on the chronicity of the condition, expectations for improvement, the role of diet and overall health, avoiding known triggers, and maintaining a healthy skin barrier.

Overall, treatment of AD involves the assessment of the skin, followed by a personalized treatment regimen that may require both rescue and maintenance or "proactive" plans. Topical corticosteroids are often used as a first-line therapy but are not without side effects. In particular, they should be minimized or avoided in areas of high sensitivity, including the face and skin folds. Crisaborole and the topical calcineurin inhibitors can be used for areas where topical corticosteroids should be avoided with a more favorable side effect profile but arguably have less efficacy as well as tolerability issues such as application site pain. Topical JAK inhibitors are strong contenders as new agents but carry a black box warning, which may introduce difficulties in counseling patients. Along with pharmaceutical treatment for AD, patients should be educated on aggravating factors and maintaining hydrated skin to prevent further epidermal barrier dysfunction (Table 7.1) (Fig. 7.2).

**Table 7.1** Selected groups of topical corticosteroids

| Potency | Corticosteroid | Forms | Percentage |
|---|---|---|---|
| Super high | Betamethasone dipropionate, augmented | Ointment (optimized), gel, lotion | 0.05 |
| Super high | Clobetasol propionate | Cream, ointment | 0.05 |
| | | Cream | 0.05 |
| | | Lotion, shampoo, aerosol spray | 0.05 |
| | | Lotion | 0.05 |
| | | Ointment | 0.05 |
| High | Fluticasone propionate | Ointment | 0.005 |
| High | Mometasone furoate | Ointment | 0.1 |
| High | Triamcinolone acetonide | Cream, ointment | 0.5 |
| Low | Desonide | Cream | 0.05 |
| | | Lotion | 0.05 |
| | | Foam | 0.05 |
| Low | Fluocinolone acetonide | Cream, solution | 0.01 |
| | | Shampoo | 0.01 |

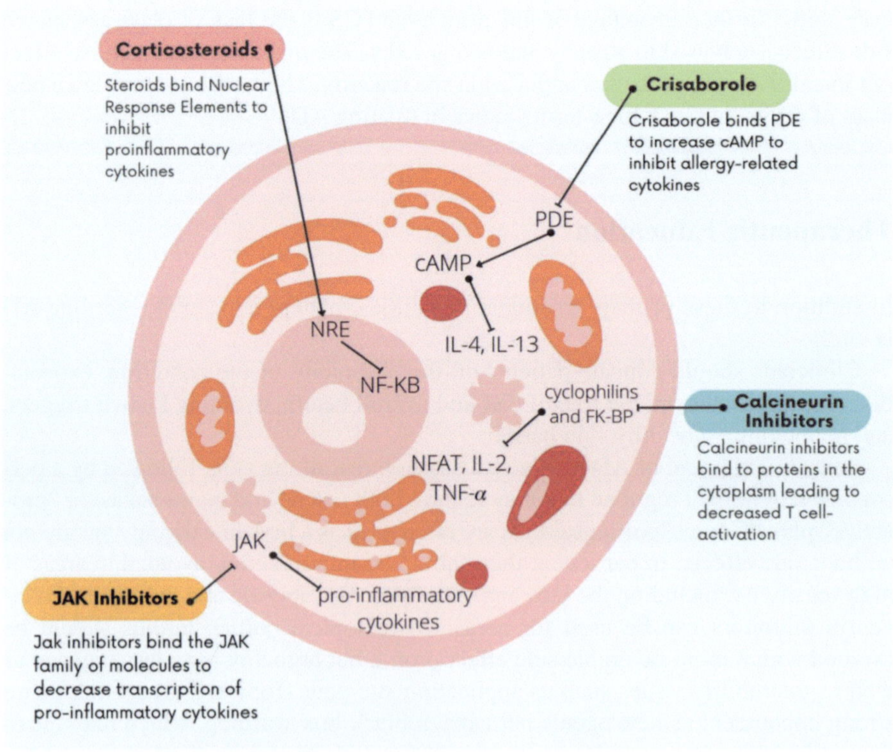


**Fig. 7.2** Pharmacological action of selected drugs

**Board Review Question Explanation**
Which of the following are possible side effects from topical corticosteroids?

A. Steroid-induced acne
B. Dermal atrophy
C. Chronic lichenification
D. Cushing's disease
E. A, C, and E
F. A, B, and D (correct)

**Explanation**
Steroid-induced acne, dermal atrophy, and even systemic effects such as Cushing's disease can all result from topical steroid use.

**Key Takeaway Points**
- The mainstays of treatment for AD are topical corticosteroids and emollients.
- Topical corticosteroids should be used with caution on the face and skin folds; non-steroidal agents may be better suited to these areas in some cases.
- Topical corticosteroids have long-term side effects including dermal atrophy, telangiectasia, and striae, making non-steroidal agents important for more longitudinal care.
- Topical JAK inhibitors show potential in effectively treating AD, but more information is still needed to fully understand these new drugs.

## Further Reading

Weston WL. Atopic dermatitis (eczema): pathogenesis, clinical manifestations, and diagnosis. In: Post TW, editor. UpToDate. Waltham, MA: UpToDate. Accessed 09 Jul 2022.

Howe W. Treatment of atopic dermatitis (eczema). In: Post TW, editor. UpToDate. Waltham, MA: UpToDate. Accessed 09 Jul 2022.

Lexicomp. Tacrolimus (topical) Drug information. In: Post TW, editor. UpToDate. Waltham, MA: UpToDate. Accessed 09 Jul 2022.

Hardinger K. Pharmacology of cyclosporine and tacrolimus. In: Post TW, editor. UpToDate. Waltham, MA: UpToDate. Accessed 09 Jul 2022.

Goldstein BG. Topical corticosteroids: use and adverse effects. In: Post TW, editor. UpToDate. Waltham, MA: UpToDate. Accessed 09 Jul 2022.

Eichenfield LF, Tom WL, Berger TG, Krol A, Paller AS, Schwarzenberger K, Bergman JN, Chamlin SL, Cohen DE, Cooper KD, Cordoro KM, Davis DM, Feldman SR, Hanifin JM, Margolis DJ, Silverman RA, Simpson EL, Williams HC, Elmets CA, Block J, Harrod CG, Smith Begolka W, Sidbury R. Guidelines of care for the management of atopic dermatitis: section 2. Management and treatment of atopic dermatitis with topical therapies. J Am Acad Dermatol. 2014;71(1):116–32. https://doi.org/10.1016/j.jaad.2014.03.023.

Frazier W, Bhardwaj N. Atopic dermatitis: diagnosis and treatment. Am Fam Physician. 2020;101(10):590–8.

Kim H, Ban J, Park MR, Kim DS, Kim HY, Han Y, Ahn K, Kim J. Effect of bathing on atopic dermatitis during the summer season. Asia Pac Allergy. 2012;2(4):269–74. https://doi.org/10.5415/apallergy.2012.2.4.269.

McDowell L, Olin B. Crisaborole: a novel nonsteroidal topical treatment for atopic dermatitis. J Pharm Technol. 2019;35(4):172–8. https://doi.org/10.1177/8755122519844507.

Google I. How much does eucrisa cost? America's #1 Prescription Medication Marketplace. https://www.usarx.com/drug/eucrisa/how-much-does-eucrisa-cost. Accessed 09 Jul 2022.

Eucrisa (crisaborole): Uses, Side Effects, Dosage & Reviews - GoodRx. GoodRx. https://www.goodrx.com/eucrisa/what-is. Accessed 09 Jul 2022.

Hwang J, Lio PA. Topical corticosteroid withdrawal ("steroid addiction"): an update of a systematic review. J Dermatol Treat. 2021;33(3):1293–8. https://doi.org/10.1080/09546634.2021.1882659.

Chang A, Robison R, Cai M, Singh AM. Natural history of food-triggered atopic dermatitis and development of immediate reactions in children. J Allergy Clin Immunol Pract. 2016;4(2):229–236.e1. https://doi.org/10.1016/j.jaip.2015.08.006.

Thompson MM, Hanifin JM. Effective therapy of childhood atopic dermatitis allays food allergy concerns. J Am Acad Dermatol. 2005;53(2 suppl 2):S214–9.

Lim NR, Lohman ME, Lio PA. The role of elimination diets in atopic dermatitis—a comprehensive review. Pediatr Dermatol. 2017;34(5):516–27. https://doi.org/10.1111/pde.13244.

Lio PA. Atopic dermatitis and food allergies: true, true and related? Arch Dis Child Educ Pract Ed. 2007;92(2):ep56–60. https://doi.org/10.1136/adc.2006.111658.

Kroodsma C. Simple vasoconstriction may be a primary antiinflammatory mechanism of topical corticosteroids. J Am Acad Dermatol. 2011;64(2 Suppl 1):AB69. https://doi.org/10.1016/j.jaad.2010.09.309. https://www.sciencedirect.com/science/article/pii/S0190962210013939

Shah VP, Peck CC, Skelly JP. `Vasoconstriction'—skin blanching—assay for glucocorticoids—a critique. Arch Dermatol. 1989;125(11):1558–61. https://doi.org/10.1001/archderm.1989.01670230100019.

Smith EW, Meyer E, Haigh JM. The human skin blanching assay for topical corticosteroid bioavailability assessment. In: Shah VP, Maibach HI, editors. Topical drug bioavailability, bioequivalence, and penetration. Boston, MA: Springer; 1993. https://doi.org/10.1007/978-1-4899-1262-6_8.

Humbert P, Guichard A. The topical corticosteroid classification called into question: towards a new approach. Exp Dermatol. 2015;24:393–5. https://doi.org/10.1111/exd.12677.

Wollenberg A, Ehmann LM. Long term treatment concepts and proactive therapy for atopic eczema. Ann Dermatol. 2012;24(3):253–60. https://doi.org/10.5021/ad.2012.24.3.253.

Chovatiya R, Paller AS. JAK inhibitors in the treatment of atopic dermatitis. J Allergy Clin Immunol. 2021;148(4):927–40. https://doi.org/10.1016/j.jaci.2021.08.009.

Fardos MI, Singh R, Perche PO, Kelly KA, Feldman SR. Evaluating topical JAK inhibitors as a treatment option for atopic dermatitis. Expert Rev Clin Immunol. 2022;18(3):221–31. https://doi.org/10.1080/1744666X.2022.1993061.

He H, Guttman-Yassky E. JAK inhibitors for atopic dermatitis: an update. Am J Clin Dermatol. 2019;20(2):181–92. https://doi.org/10.1007/s40257-018-0413-2. Erratum in: Am J Clin Dermatol. 2019 Jan 10.

Rodrigues MA, Torres T. JAK/STAT inhibitors for the treatment of atopic dermatitis. J Dermatolog Treat. 2020 Feb;31(1):33–40. https://doi.org/10.1080/09546634.2019.1577549.

Cotter DG, Schairer D, Eichenfield L. Emerging therapies for atopic dermatitis: JAK inhibitors. J Am Acad Dermatol. 2018 Mar;78(3 Suppl 1):S53–62. https://doi.org/10.1016/j.jaad.2017.12.019.

Nezamololama N, Fieldhouse K, Metzger K, Gooderham M. Emerging systemic JAK inhibitors in the treatment of atopic dermatitis: a review of abrocitinib, baricitinib, and upadacitinib. Drugs Context. 2020;9:2020-8-5. https://doi.org/10.7573/dic.2020-8-5.

Traidl S, Freimooser S, Werfel T. Janus kinase inhibitors for the therapy of atopic dermatitis. Allergol Select. 2021;5:293–304. https://doi.org/10.5414/ALX02272E.

Thom H, Cheng V, Keeney E, Neary MP, Eccleston A, Zang C, Cappelleri JC, Cha A, Thyssen JP. Matching-adjusted indirect comparison of Crisaborole Ointment 2% vs. Topical Calcineurin inhibitors in the treatment of patients with mild-to-moderate atopic dermatitis. Dermatol Ther (Heidelb). 2022;12(1):185–94. https://doi.org/10.1007/s13555-021-00646-1.

Gutfreund K, Bienias W, Szewczyk A, Kaszuba A. Topical calcineurin inhibitors in dermatology. Part I: properties, method and effectiveness of drug use. Postepy Dermatol Alergol. 2013;30(3):165–9. https://doi.org/10.5114/pdia.2013.35619.

Paller AS, Fölster-Holst R, Chen SC, Diepgen TL, Elmets C, Margolis DJ, Pollock BH. No evidence of increased cancer incidence in children using topical tacrolimus for atopic dermatitis. J Am Acad Dermatol. 2020;83(2):375–81. https://doi.org/10.1016/j.jaad.2020.03.075.

Milingou M, Antille C, Sorg O, Saurat JH, Lübbe J. Alcohol intolerance and facial flushing in patients treated with topical tacrolimus. Arch Dermatol. 2004;140(12):1542–4. https://doi.org/10.1001/archderm.140.12.1542-b.

Carr WW. Topical calcineurin inhibitors for atopic dermatitis: review and treatment recommendations. Paediatr Drugs. 2013;15(4):303–10. https://doi.org/10.1007/s40272-013-0013-9.

# Chapter 8
# Treatment of AD with Ruxolitinib

**Bo Young Chung, Faye Orcales, Alexander Ildardashty, Tina Bhutani, and Wilson Liao**

**Case Title** A 24-year-old female with atopic dermatitis on the face.

**Case**

A 24-year-old female presented to the clinic with a red rash on the face. Symptoms included severe itching. Her symptoms started when she was 2 years old and have continued until now. At first, there were skin lesions on flexor parts of the arms and legs. In the recent 2–3 years, there has been a tendency for lesions to persist only on the face. Her other medical issues included asthma. The only known family history is in her father, who has atopic dermatitis.

The patient was using desonide cream for about 10 years intermittently when the facial skin rash worsened. She is worried about the side effects of topical corticosteroids and doesn't want to use desonide 0.05% cream anymore. She previously tried to use tacrolimus ointment and pimecrolimus cream for treating her facial skin lesions. However, due to experiencing burning and stinging, she stopped using tacrolimus ointment and pimecrolimus cream.

On physical examination, ill-defined, erythematous plaques were noted on the forehead and periocular areas with excoriations and lichenification, affecting about

B. Y. Chung
Department of Dermatology, University of California, San Francisco, San Francisco, CA, USA

Department of Dermatology, Hallym University Kangnam Sacred Heart Hospital, Hallym University College of Medicine, Seoul, South Korea

F. Orcales · T. Bhutani · W. Liao (✉)
Department of Dermatology, University of California, San Francisco, San Francisco, CA, USA
e-mail: Faye.Orcales@ucsf.edu; tina.bhutani@ucsf.edu; wilson.liao@ucsf.edu

A. Ildardashty
Sackler School of Medicine, Tel Aviv University, Tel Aviv, Israel



N. Brownstone et al. (eds.), *Clinical Cases in Atopic Dermatitis*, Clinical Cases in Dermatology, https://doi.org/10.1007/978-3-031-52147-8_8

1% of body surface area. Folds in the skin below the lower eyelid (Dennie-Morgan infraorbital folds) were observed. The skin on her whole body displayed dryness.

**Board Review Question**

Based on the clinical description, which topical agent would be the best option for treating the facial skin lesions of this patient?

A. Calcipotriene cream
B. Pimecrolimus cream
C. Tacrolimus ointment
D. Triamcinolone 0.5% cream
E. Ruxolitinib 1.5% cream

## Main Text

Topical agents such as corticosteroids and topical calcineurin inhibitors are commonly used for mild to moderate AD as the first line of treatment [1]. However, cases of withdrawal, steroid rebound, and numerous side effects have generated phobia toward topical corticosteroid use. Topical calcineurin inhibitors also tend to have a high rate of application site reactions (e.g., stinging). For many years, the lack of a safe yet effective treatment for AD has warranted a need for more comprehensive treatments.

In recent years, Janus kinase (JAK) inhibition has shown potential as a novel therapeutic for AD. Numerous studies indicate that the increased production of T helper 2 (Th2)-type immune-inducing factors is a significant causal factor for AD. Th2 produces various cytokines such as interleukin-4 (IL-4) and interleukin-13 (IL-13). Expression of these cytokines' receptors was shown to have direct effects on pruritus and skin barrier dysfunction [2].

The JAK-STAT pathway is a significant signaling pathway downstream of many Th2 cytokine receptors. The JAK-STAT pathway is activated when a ligand, such as a cytokine or growth factor, binds to a cell surface receptor. This leads to the activation of JAK enzymes, which then phosphorylate STAT proteins, leading to their dimerization and translocation to the nucleus. In the nucleus, the dimerized STAT proteins bind to specific DNA sequences and regulate gene expression.

Ruxolitinib works by inhibiting the activity of JAK enzymes, specifically JAK1 and JAK2. When these enzymes are inhibited, they are unable to phosphorylate STAT proteins, leading to a disruption of the JAK-STAT signaling pathway and a reduction in inflammation. This is thought to be mediated through the suppression of the production of pro-inflammatory cytokines, such as IL-4 and IL-13, which are involved in the development and maintenance of inflammation in AD [3].

In addition to inhibiting the activity of JAK enzymes, ruxolitinib may also have additional mechanisms of action. For example, it has been shown to inhibit the production of matrix metalloproteinases (MMPs), which are enzymes that break down extracellular matrix proteins and are involved in the development of skin inflammation [4]. Ruxolitinib may also have anti-oxidative and anti-apoptotic effects, which may contribute to its anti-inflammatory properties [5].

In conclusion, ruxolitinib works by inhibiting the activity of JAK enzymes, specifically JAK1 and JAK2, which disrupts the JAK-STAT signaling pathway and leads to a reduction in inflammation. This is thought to be mediated through the suppression of the production of pro-inflammatory cytokines and may be enhanced by additional mechanisms of action, such as the inhibition of MMP production and anti-oxidative and anti-apoptotic effects.

## Efficacy and Safety

Ruxolitinib has undergone clinical trials to examine its efficacy and safety for treatment of atopic dermatitis (AD) (Table 8.1). A double-blind, 8-week, phase II, dose-ranging study for 307 adult patients with AD reported that ruxolitinib (RUX) cream showed increasing improvement over time and with higher concentrations [6]. 1.5% RUX cream twice daily (BID) achieved a significantly greater mean percentage improvement from baseline in EASI score and Investigator's Global Assessment (IGA) response versus vehicle at week 4. Significant itch reduction was observed as early as within 36 h of initiation of treatment with 1.5% RUX cream BID versus vehicle and was sustained over the 12 weeks of treatment.

The two identically designed vehicle-controlled, double-blind, 8-week, phase III studies (TRuE AD1, TRuE AD2) for adolescent and adult patient with AD showed that significantly more patients achieved IGA treatment success with 0.75% RUX and 1.5% RUX versus vehicle [7]. Significantly greater reductions in itch versus vehicle were observed within 12 h of the first application of 1.5% RUX cream, and further reductions were observed over 8 weeks.

In these three studies, RUX cream was well tolerated, and systemic safety concerns associated with oral JAK inhibitors were not observed [6–8]. In phase II study, application site pain was the most common treatment-related AE in any RUX cream group (0.15% QD, 2.0%; 1.5% QD, 3.9%; 1.5% BID, 2.0%) and was also shown in vehicle group (3.8%). No significant laboratory changes were reported. Two phase III studies showed similar safety profiles with phase II study. Application site reactions were rare and lower with RUX cream groups versus vehicle group (vehicle, 4.4%; 0.75% RUX, 0.6%; 1.5% RUX, 0.8%). Regarding pharmacokinetics analysis, overall bioavailability of RUX cream is low, and the average steady-state trough plasma concentrations at its highest strength (1.5% cream BID) are well below that required for clinically relevant systemic pharmacological activity [8]. Ruxolitinib was eventually given FDA approval in September of 2021 and represents a novel approach for targeting AD [9].

**Table 8.1** Clinical trials of ruxolitinib cream for treatment of atopic dermatitis

| Authors and year | Patients | Study design | Main results |
|---|---|---|---|
| Kim et al. (2020) [7] | Adolescent and adult patient with atopic dermatitis (aged ≥12 years with AD for ≥2 years, IGA score of 2/3, 3–20% BSA) | The two identically designed vehicle-controlled, double-blind, 8-week, phase III studies (TRuE AD1, TRuE AD2)<br>631 and 618 patients were randomized (2:2:1) to topical treatment with ruxolitinib 0.75% BID, ruxolitinib 1.5% BID, or vehicle cream. After the 8-week study period, in the 44-week extension study period, patients initially randomized to the vehicle treatment were randomized (1:1) to topical ruxolitinib 0.75% or 1.5% cream BID, whereas those initially randomized to a ruxolitinib cream remained on the same regimen | – Efficacy: 631 and 577 patients were analyzed for efficacy. Significantly more patients achieved Investigator's global assessment treatment success with 0.75% ruxolitinib and 1.5% ruxolitinib versus vehicle. Significantly greater reductions in itch versus vehicle were observed within 12 h of the first application of 1.5% ruxolitinib cream, and further reductions were observed over 8 weeks<br>– Safety: Ruxolitinib cream showed an unremarkable safety profile. Application site reactions were infrequent with ruxolitinib cream |
| Papp et al. (2021) [6] | 307 adult patients with atopic dermatitis (aged 18–70 years with AD for ≥2 years, IGA score of 2/3, 3–20% BSA) | A double-blind, 8-week, phase II, dose-ranging study<br>Randomized (1:1:1:1:1) to topical treatment with the following creams: Ruxolitinib 0.15% once daily (QD), ruxolitinib 0.5% QD, ruxolitinib 1.5% QD, ruxolitinib 1.5% twice daily (BID), vehicle BID, or active control (triamcinolone 0.1% BID) | – Efficacy: All concentrations of ruxolitinib cream demonstrated the improvement in the signs and symptoms of AD versus vehicle. 1.5% RUX cream BID achieved a significantly greater mean percentage improvement from baseline in EASI score and IGA response versus vehicle at week 4. Significant itch reduction was observed as early as within 36 h of initiation of treatment with 1.5% RUX cream BID versus vehicle and was sustained over the 12 weeks of treatment. Although these were not statistically significant, 1.5% RUX cream BID reported greater improvement in EASI score and IGA response compared with triamcinolone at week 4<br>– Safety: Ruxolitinib cream was well tolerated with no serious side effects reported |

| | | | |
|---|---|---|---|
| Bissonnette et al. (2022) [14] | 41 AD patients (ages 12–65, IGA ≥2, and ≥ 25% affected BSA) | Open-label, maximum-use, phase I, 56-day study Patients applied 1.5% ruxolitinib cream on baseline-identified lesions twice daily for 28 days. Cream was applied only to active lesions for an additional 28 days | – Efficacy: At day 56, 94.6% of patients achieved ≥75% improvement in the EASI<br>– Safety: Maximum use of ruxolitinib cream was generally tolerable. 13/41 (~1/3) patients experienced a treatment-emergent adverse event. 4/41 (~10%) patients experienced a treatment-related adverse event |

*AD* atopic dermatitis, *IGA* investigator's global assessment, *BSA* body surface area, *EASI* eczema area and severity index

**Board Review Question Explanation**

Based on the clinical description, which topical agent would be the best option for treating the facial skin lesions of this patient?

A. Calcipotriene cream
B. Pimecrolimus cream
C. Tacrolimus ointment
D. Triamcinolone 0.5% cream
E. Ruxolitinib 1.5% cream (correct)

**Explanation**

Atopic dermatitis is a common chronic inflammatory skin disorder associated with significant itch. The major clinical features of AD are pruritus, erythematous and ill-defined eruption or lichenification involving the flexural areas/skin creases, xerosis, and a personal or family history of atopy (asthma, allergic rhinitis, atopic dermatitis). Associated characteristics include stigmata such as Dennie-Morgan lines [10]. AD has variable rates of remission, with some patients developing or continuing symptoms into adulthood. The pruritus is a challenging symptom of AD, which can be refractory to conventional treatments for AD such as topical corticosteroids or topical calcineurin inhibitors. This patient has AD based on the clinical findings.

This patient has used a low-potency corticosteroid agent (desonide 0.05% cream) for clearing her flare intermittently for a long period. Topical corticosteroids are a conventional therapeutic method for AD. However, we should consider potential side effects such as skin atrophy, striae, and purpura when topical corticosteroids are used for prolonged periods in sensitive areas such as the face. This AD patient is presenting mainly with facial lesions. Thus, triamcinolone 0.5% cream (medium-potency corticosteroid) is not appropriate for the treatment of this case.

Topical calcineurin inhibitors (tacrolimus, pimecrolimus) have been approved for AD treatments since 2006. The treatment efficacy of tacrolimus ointment is similar to that of a low- to medium-potency corticosteroid. Topical calcineurin inhibitors avoid some of the side effects of topical corticosteroids such as skin thinning, striae, and purpura [11]. However, application site reactions such as burning and stinging sensation are common with calcineurin inhibitors [12]. These adverse effects can reduce the patient adherence to topical calcineurin inhibitors.

Calcipotriene cream is a vitamin D analog, which regulates the epidermal hyperproliferation and local immune system including Th1 cytokine production [13]. Vitamin D analogs are usually used for treatment of psoriasis. Vitamin D analogs do not elicit skin atrophy. However, the most common side effect of vitamin D analog is irritation. Thus, vitamin D analogs may not be suitable for sensitive areas of the skin, particularly the face.

Recent phase I, II, and III studies for topical ruxolitinib (RUX) cream in patients with AD demonstrated that topical RUX cream has rapid and sustained efficacy for AD [6, 7, 14]. Notably, pruritus has been well controlled by RUX cream in AD. Furthermore, RUX cream is well tolerated and safe without significant side effects. Therefore, RUX 1.5% cream is a safe therapeutic approach for particularly sensitive areas such as the face, axilla, and inguinal areas with considerable efficacy for itching. Based on these, RUX cream is the best option for this mild AD case with facial involvement.

**Key Takeaway Points**

- Conventional treatments for mild to moderate AD include topical corticosteroids and topical calcineurin inhibitors. Long-term use of topical corticosteroids is associated with side effects such as skin thinning, striae, and purpura. Topical calcineurin inhibitors may lead to application site reactions.
- Ruxolitinib cream is a topical agent that works as a JAK inhibitor.
- In clinical trials, 1.5% ruxolitinib cream is shown to have a significant improvement on symptoms of AD including itching, without significant side effects.

## References

1. Chovatiya R, Paller AS. JAK inhibitors in the treatment of atopic dermatitis. J Allergy Clin Immunol. 2021;148(4):927–40.
2. Nakashima C, Yanagihara S, Otsuka A. Innovation in the treatment of atopic dermatitis: emerging topical and oral Janus kinase inhibitors. Allergol Int. 2022;71(1):40–6.
3. Traidl S, Freimooser S, Werfel T. Janus kinase inhibitors for the therapy of atopic dermatitis. Allergol Select. 2021;5:293–304. https://doi.org/10.5414/ALX02272E.
4. Liu GM, Zhang LJ, Fu JZ, Liang WT, Cheng ZY, Bai P, Bian YS, Wan JS. Regulation of Ruxolitinib on matrix metalloproteinase in JAK2V617F positive myeloproliferative neoplasms cells. Zhonghua Xue Ye Xue Za Zhi. 2017;38(2):140–5. https://doi.org/10.3760/cma.j.issn.0253-2727.2017.02.011.
5. Elli EM, Baratè C, Mendicino F, Palandri F, Palumbo GA. Mechanisms underlying the anti-inflammatory and immunosuppressive activity of Ruxolitinib. Front Oncol. 2019;9:1186. https://doi.org/10.3389/fonc.2019.01186.
6. Papp K, Szepietowski JC, Kircik L, Toth D, Eichenfield LF, Leung DYM, et al. Efficacy and safety of ruxolitinib cream for the treatment of atopic dermatitis: results from 2 phase 3, randomized, double-blind studies. J Am Acad Dermatol. 2021;85(4):863–72.
7. Kim BS, Howell MD, Sun K, Papp K, Nasir A, Kuligowski ME, et al. Treatment of atopic dermatitis with ruxolitinib cream (JAK1/JAK2 inhibitor) or triamcinolone cream. J Allergy Clin Immunol. 2020;145(2):572–82.
8. Gong X, Chen X, Kuligowski ME, Liu X, Liu X, Cimino E, et al. Pharmacokinetics of Ruxolitinib in patients with atopic dermatitis treated with Ruxolitinib cream: data from phase II and III studies. Am J Clin Dermatol. 2021;22(4):555–66.
9. Owji S, Caldas SA, Ungar B. Management of Atopic Dermatitis: clinical utility of Ruxolitinib. J Asthma Allergy. 2022;15:1527–37. https://doi.org/10.2147/JAA.S342051.
10. Weidinger S, Novak N. Atopic dermatitis. Lancet. 2016;387(10023):1109–22.
11. Fukaya M, Sato K, Sato M, Kimata H, Fujisawa S, Dozono H, Yoshizawa J, Minaguchi S. Topical steroid addiction in atopic dermatitis. Drug Healthc Patient Saf. 2014;6:131–8. https://doi.org/10.2147/dhps.s6920.
12. Czarnecka-Operacz M, Jenerowicz D. Topical calcineurin inhibitors in the treatment of atopic dermatitis – an update on safety issues. JDDG. J Dtsch Dermatol Ges. 2012;10:167–72.
13. van de Kerkhof PC. Biological activity of vitamin D analogues in the skin, with special reference to antipsoriatic mechanisms. Br J Dermatol. 1995;132(5):675–82.
14. Bissonnette R, Call RS, Raoof T, Zhu Z, Yeleswaram S, Gong X, Lee M. A maximum-use trial of Ruxolitinib cream in adolescents and adults with atopic dermatitis. Am J Clin Dermatol. 2022;23(3):355–64.

# Chapter 9
# Treatment of Atopic Dermatitis with Phototherapy

**Rachel K. Greene and Mio Nakamura**

### Case

A 22-year-old female with a 3-year history of atopic dermatitis presents for a follow-up visit to the dermatologist. She reports feeling itchy at night, which interferes with her sleep. Her skin is sensitive to certain detergents, lotions, and fabrics such as wool. Currently, she is using topical steroids for the body, topical tacrolimus for the face, and antihistamines for the pruritus. Recently, she completed an 8-week course of oral corticosteroids with only short-term relief. Physical exam reveals diffuse erythematous plaques with excoriations and lichenification on her face, neck, trunk, antecubital fossae, hands, and popliteal fossae. The patient is not using any form of birth control and is considering becoming pregnant in the next year. She works from home and has a flexible work schedule.

**Board Review Question**
At this time, what therapy would you recommend to the patient?

A. Trimethoprim–sulfamethoxazole
B. Narrowband ultraviolet B (NB-UVB) phototherapy
C. Continue current regimen
D. Methotrexate
E. Dilute bleach baths and emollients

## Overview

Atopic dermatitis (AD) is a common inflammatory skin disease characterized by a disrupted skin barrier leading to immune activation. Due to the chronic relapsing nature of this disease, management includes both treatment of acute flares and a

R. K. Greene · M. Nakamura (✉)
Department of Dermatology, University of Michigan, Ann Arbor, MI, USA
e-mail: mionak@med.umich.edu



N. Brownstone et al. (eds.), *Clinical Cases in Atopic Dermatitis*, Clinical Cases in Dermatology, https://doi.org/10.1007/978-3-031-52147-8_9

long-term maintenance regimen. While topical corticosteroids and topical steroid-sparing agents are the first-line treatment of AD, systemic treatment or phototherapy may be needed for adequate disease control in moderate to severe cases.

Phototherapy was first reported as a dermatologic treatment modality in 1925. William Goeckerman formulated a regimen consisting of crude coal tar followed by broadband ultraviolet B (BB-UVB) for severe or refractory psoriasis [1]. In the 1920s, AD was observed to improve in sea–air climates during the summer, but it was not until 1948 when the efficacy of BB-UVB using carbon arc lamps was discovered to be an effective treatment for AD. Several decades later in 1978, a publication from Massachusetts General Hospital reported clearance of refractory AD with oral administration of 8-methoxypsoralen followed by ultraviolet A irradiation (PUVA) [2, 3].

In this chapter, we will discuss the mechanism of action of phototherapy and review the safety and efficacy of broadband UVB (BB-UVB), NB-UVB, Goeckerman regimen (coal tar and UVB), excimer laser, psoralen and UVA (PUVA), and combination therapy with phototherapy for AD. Lastly, home phototherapy will be discussed.

## Mechanism of Action of Phototherapy

Phototherapy is effective for the treatment of AD primarily due to its immunosuppressive effects. UV light directly targets T-cell-mediated inflammation and decreases interleukin (IL)-17 and IL-22 in the skin [4], which are pathogenic in AD. Langerhans cells and dermal dendritic cells are also sensitive to UVB, which can reduce the expression of ICAM-1 and other adhesion molecules, causing a reduction in antigen-presenting cell function to the effector T cells [5]. UV radiation may also induce keratinocyte-derived antimicrobial peptides that prevent skin colonization by pathogens [6]. The interplay of photobiology pathways in AD is not completely understood and requires further investigation.

## When to Recommend Phototherapy

Phototherapy is an effective treatment option for patients with AD who have failed topical treatments. UVB phototherapy is a safe option that has no internal side effects. Therefore, it can be used in pediatric patients and women who are pregnant, nursing, or of childbearing potential [7, 8]. Phototherapy should not be administered to patients with erythrodermic AD, as UV light can worsen erythroderma. Phototherapy should be avoided in patients with photosensitizing disorders such as xeroderma pigmentosum and porphyria [9]. Patients with AD affecting the scalp or intertriginous areas may not benefit from phototherapy, as the UV light cannot penetrate effectively in these areas. Safe administration of phototherapy requires standing still within the booth for a prescribed amount of time. Therefore, young children or patients with mobility issues such as wheelchair-bound patients or those requiring walkers may not be good candidates for phototherapy. Patients must also be able to tolerate wearing eye protection throughout the duration of phototherapy treatments. Furthermore, phototherapy requires special equipment and trained staff to administer the treatment and is typically performed in-office. Phototherapy requires a significant time commitment and may disrupt the patient's school or work. Patients without reliable transportation to and from the office may also be inappropriate for phototherapy. For certain patients, home phototherapy may be an option to overcome these challenges [10]. Lastly, insurance coverage for phototherapy should be confirmed prior to initiating treatment. Treatments may become cost-prohibitive for some patients, given phototherapy is often prescribed as a long-term maintenance regimen for treatment of AD.

## UVB Phototherapy

### *Dosing*

The initial dose of UVB is determined by Fitzpatrick skin phototype (FSP) or minimal erythema dose (MED) (Table 9.1) [11]. MED is defined as the lowest UV dose that produces a perceived area of erythema on the skin [12]. The dose is increased at each subsequent visit as tolerated up to a maximum dose of 2000–5000 mJ/cm$^2$ for NB-UVB depending on FSP (Table 9.1) [11]. Treatments are administered three times per week initially and may be gradually decreased after stable improvement has been reached, typically after 12–16 weeks. Table 9.2 shows the dosing protocol for missed treatment sessions, as the dose must be decreased after missing 12 or more days of treatment.

### *Efficacy of NB-UVB (311–313 nm)*

Several studies have demonstrated the efficacy and long-term benefit of NB-UVB for patients with AD. NB-UVB has been shown to improve AD clinical scores and reduce necessity for topical steroids [13–15]. After completing treatment with NB-UVB, patients with AD may achieve clinical remission for up to 6 months [16]. In another study, 12 patients received NB-UVB phototherapy three times weekly for up to 12 weeks. All patients achieved at least a 50% reduction in the scoring of atopic dermatitis index (SCORAD) [17].

The effectiveness of NB-UVB has also been evaluated in children. A retrospective study examined the effects of NB-UVB on children with severe AD. Out of 50 children, 40% achieved minimal residual activity or clearance [18]. The median length of remission was 3 months [18]. Another study evaluated 30 children with moderate to severe AD who received NB-UVB phototherapy twice weekly for 24 weeks [19]. The baseline mean SCORAD was greater than 30, and after completing treatment, the mean SCORAD significantly decreased to 7.82 [19]. While NB-UVB can be beneficial in the pediatric population, it may be limited by compliance, age, and maturity, as the child must be able to follow directions for safe administration [18, 20].

**Table 9.1** Ultraviolet B (UVB) dosing protocols

| Narrowband UVB dosing protocol based on Fitzpatrick skin type | | | |
|---|---|---|---|
| Fitzpatrick skin type | Initial dose (mJ/cm$^2$) | Dose increments (mJ/cm$^2$) | Maximum dose (mJ/cm$^2$) |
| I | 130 | 15 | 2000 |
| II | 220 | 25 | 2000 |
| III | 260 | 40 | 3000 |
| IV | 330 | 45 | 3000 |
| V | 350 | 60 | 5000 |
| VI | 400 | 65 | 5000 |

| Narrowband UVB dosing protocol based on minimal erythema dose (MED) | |
|---|---|
| Treatment session | Recommendation |
| Initial session | 50% of MED |
| 1–20 | Increase dose by 10% of initial MED |

**Table 9.2** Ultraviolet B (UVB) missed treatment protocols

| Narrowband UVB missed treatment protocol | |
|---|---|
| Duration between treatment | Recommendation |
| 1–7 days | Increase dose per protocol |
| 8–11 days | Continue current dose |
| 12–20 days | Decrease by 25% |
| 21–27 days | Decrease by 50% |
| Greater than 28 days | Restart at initial dose |

## *Efficacy of Broadband UVB (290–320 nm)*

BB-UVB is one of the oldest forms of phototherapy for treating AD and is no longer widely available [21]. However, it remains an important phototherapy modality, as some patients with AD may better tolerate BB-UVB over NB-UVB. In one study, 17 patients with AD were treated with BB-UVB (0.5–1 MED) compared with visible light [22]. The regimen comprised of treating half the body with BB-UVB and the other half with visible light for 8 weeks. AD lesions improved considerably in areas treated by BB-UVB compared to visible light in 13 patients. The same study investigated the efficacy of 0.8 MED versus 0.4 MED of BB-UVB in 25 patients and found no significant difference in efficacy [22]. This supports the idea that providers may start BB-UVB at lower doses and gradually increase the dosing if the disease is refractory.

## *Safety*

Adverse effects of UVB phototherapy are mild but should be considered before initiating treatment. Acute side effects include erythema, itching, burning, and stinging. The risk of burning is greater with BB-UVB compared to NB-UVB. Eye protection must be worn to avoid the risk of keratitis. During a treatment session, overheating and perspiration caused by the phototherapy unit may cause discomfort to the patient. These side effects may cause an AD flare. Air-conditioned NB-UVB regimens can help overcome these issues and help with patient adherence and tolerability [23]. The immunosuppressive properties of UVB may cause possible reactivation of the herpes simplex or varicella zoster virus [24] but are not associated with an increased risk of other cutaneous infections. Long-term effects of UVB phototherapy include tanning and photoaging. Cumulative exposure to UVB causes actinic damage regardless of the UVB source.

While UVB phototherapy is safe for pregnant women, some studies show that high cumulative doses of UVB treatment may decrease serum folic acid levels, which can lead to neural tube defects [25–27]. It is important to note that other studies have not been able to reproduce this statement and this issue is widely debated [28]. It may be beneficial to supplement pregnant women and women of childbearing potential with folic acid while receiving phototherapy [29].

## *Goeckerman Regimen (Coal Tar and UVB)*

Goeckerman therapy consists of daily UVB exposure to the skin followed by application of crude coal tar (CCT) under occlusion for at least 4 h each day [30, 31]. In a small study, five patients with that five patients with chronic, severe AD who were unresponsive to BB-UVB, NB-UVB, or systemic immunosuppressants were treated daily with BB-UVB followed by CCT and topical corticosteroids in an outpatient setting for an average of 27 days [31]. All the patients demonstrated a significant improvement with a reduction of the baseline SCORAD by at least 75%. Patients remained in remission for 5–12 months [31]. While the Goeckerman regimen is highly effective, the topical preparation of the CCT can be messy and malodorous. Some patients can experience worsening itching caused by the warmth and occlusion, as well as folliculitis. Other disadvantages include increased cost to patients for inpatient or day treatment admission and time commitment [32].

## *Excimer Laser (308 nm)*

The excimer laser is a targeted UVB phototherapy using a monochromatic beam of light. Currently, it is approved by the Food and Drug Administration (FDA) for the treatment of psoriasis and vitiligo [33]. The excimer laser is advantageous for patients with localized disease and avoids full-body irradiation. In a study of 15 patients with AD involving less than 20% body surface area, mean severity scores were significantly lower after twice weekly treatments for 4 weeks [34]. Another study showed that the excimer laser is effective for treating recalcitrant hand and foot dermatitis [35]. Excimer laser is a beneficial treatment modality for localized dermatitis in adults and children [36]. The acute side effects of the excimer laser are similar to UVB phototherapy [35].

# PUVA

## *Dosing*

PUVA is a type of photochemotherapy combining UVA with a psoralen, 8-methoxypsoralen (8-MOP), or methoxsalen. 8-MOP can be taken orally (systemic PUVA) or applied topically in a cream or bath (topical and bath PUVA) [3]. The dosage of oral 8-MOP is weight based at 0.4–0.6 mg/kg to be taken 1–2 h before UVA exposure [37]. Bath PUVA includes 20–30 min of bathing in warm water containing 8-MOP at a concentration of 0.5–3 mg/L followed by UVA exposure. Patients with localized disease such as hand eczema may use topical PUVA in which topical psoralen is applied to the affected areas, followed by UVA exposure 30–60 min later [21]. UVA treatments are administered 2–3 times per week, at least 48 h apart. The starting dose is determined by FSP, and if no erythema is noted between treatments, the UVA dose may be increased by 0.5–1.5 J/cm$^2$ depending on FSP (Table 9.3) [21]. Table 9.4 shows the missed dosing protocol for PUVA.

**Table 9.3** PUVA dosing protocol by Fitzpatrick skin type

| Fitzpatrick skin type | Initial dose (J/cm$^2$) | Dose increments (J/cm$^2$) | Maximum dose (J/cm$^2$) |
|---|---|---|---|
| I | 1.5 | 0.5 | 5 |
| II | 2.5 | 0.5 | 8 |
| III | 3.5 | 0.5–1.0 | 12 |
| IV | 4.5 | 1.0 | 14 |
| V | 5.5 | 1.0 | 16 |
| VI | 6.5 | 1.0–1.5 | 20 |

**Table 9.4** PUVA missed treatment protocol

| Number of missed treatments | Recommendation |
|---|---|
| 1 | Repeat previous dose and then continue previous increments |
| 2 | Repeat previous dose |
| 3 | Treat at second to last dose |
| 4–6 | Give 50% of last dose |
| Greater than 2 weeks | Consult the clinician |

## *Efficacy of PUVA*

Systemic PUVA is efficacious for the treatment of AD. One study of 15 patients with severe AD showed 99% improvement of AD in all patients after an average of 36 treatments [3]. This study also found that PUVA is more effective than UVB, and long-term treatment is needed to maintain clearance.

In another study, 15 children with AD were treated with PUVA for an average of 16 weeks [38]. Clinical remission was achieved in nine of the patients [38]. Interestingly, the treatment allowed resumption of normal growth in these children who were previously growing poorly [38]. This may be secondary to the improvement of the severe AD. Another study evaluated 53 children with AD who were unresponsive to topical corticosteroids and emollients. Seventy-four percent of the patients achieved greater than 90% clearance after an average of 9 weeks of PUVA treatment [39].

## *Safety*

Although PUVA is effective, it is less commonly used compared to UVB phototherapy due to the side effect profile of systemic PUVA and the logistical requirements of topical/bath PUVA. The most common short-term side effect of systemic PUVA is nausea. Taking 8-MOP with a meal may reduce or prevent nausea. Sun protective eye gear should be worn for 24 h after taking 8-MOP [40]. Erythema following PUVA is delayed compared to that of UVB, occurring 48–96 h after exposure [41]. Side effects of PUVA include skin hyperpigmentation, lentigines, photoaging, and long-term carcinogenic risk (see below). Patients with photosensitizing diseases such as xeroderma pigmentosum, lupus, or porphyria and pregnant or lactating women should not be treated with PUVA [9].

## Home Phototherapy

Home-based phototherapy (HBPT) allows patients to overcome barriers to in-office phototherapy. Travel, co-pays, and missed school or work due to frequent clinic visits can limit access to in-office treatment. HBPT can increase treatment compliance and reduce logistical burden on patients. Various types of devices are available including full-body or half-body panels, hand/foot booths, and handheld devices. During the COVID-19 pandemic, HBPT was a useful treatment option; it allowed patients to continue treatments at home and decrease the potential spread of the virus [42]. During the pandemic, a retrospective study found that over 88% of patients felt their disease improved since starting home phototherapy [43]. For AD, there have been no studies examining the safety or efficacy of HBPT versus in-office phototherapy [11]. In psoriasis, the effects of home phototherapy are widely studied, and some studies suggest that HBPT may not be as effective as in-office phototherapy [44, 45]. However, the landmark PLUTO trial assessing the cost-effectiveness of HBPT versus outpatient phototherapy concluded that HBPT is a cost-effective treatment option for patients and is equally as effective as office-based treatment [10, 46].

While HBPT is a safe treatment option, patients should be educated on proper dosing to avoid side effects such as burning [47]. Most devices require a code provided by a physician and have safety features such as key-locked switches, timers to limit length of treatment, and a system that allows only a set number of treatments before requiring follow-up with a prescribing provider.

## Combination Therapy

Systemic and topical agents may be used in conjunction with phototherapy and are commonly prescribed in clinical practice. The goal of combination therapy is to improve efficacy and reduce side effects. One study of 844 AD patients found that the majority (70%) of patients with AD required less use of topical corticosteroids during the 12-month window after finishing NB-UVB compared to the 12-month window before starting the treatment [61]. In a study of 26 children with AD, the combination of topical pimecrolimus 1% cream and NB-UVB did not show superior efficacy to either monotherapy [48]. Another study evaluated the combination of NB-UVB and UVA and found that the combination was not superior to NB-UVB alone [49]. A study found that combining NB-UVB and dupilumab resulted in faster remission of severe AD in the first few weeks of dupilumab therapy [50]. A study by Gori et al. also showed improvement of AD with NB-UVB in one patient who failed dupilumab monotherapy [51]. Overall, studies investigating combination therapy regimens using phototherapy for the treatment of AD are limited. Further studies are needed to better understand the safety and efficacy of combining phototherapy with other treatment modalities for AD.

## Risk of Skin Cancer from Phototherapy

The risk of skin cancer from phototherapy is a relevant topic to clinicians and patients. A retrospective study evaluated 925 patients with AD who received NB-UVB, BB-UVB, or concurrent UVA plus BB-UVB and found no increased risk of basal cell carcinoma (BCC), squamous cell carcinoma (SCC), or melanoma, except in patients who had a history of taking immunosuppressive therapy [52]. There have not been additional studies specifically investigating skin cancer risk in AD patients. The evidence summarized below is mostly based on studies in psoriasis patients.

A study consisting of more than 3800 patients found no significant association between NB-UVB treatment and BCC, SCC, and melanoma [53]. Patients who were previously treated with PUVA and then treated with NB-UVB had a slight increase in BCCs [53]. Another cross-sectional study of 100 age- and sex-matched patients treated with NB-UVB revealed no cases of melanoma [54]. Another cross-sectional study assessed the risk of skin cancer in psoriasis patients treated with NB-UVB or BB-UVB. The skin cancer risk increased with the number of treatments when controlling for age [55]. More longitudinal studies are needed to examine the relationship between NB-UVB and skin cancer.

For PUVA, long-term studies have shown a dose-related increase in incidence of nonmelanoma skin cancers in Caucasian psoriasis patients who are exposed to a high cumulative dose of oral PUVA. In a 30-year follow-up study of more than 1300 patients with severe psoriasis treated with PUVA, the incidence of SCC was 30 times higher in patients who received more than 500 treatments of PUVA compared to patients receiving lower doses [56]. Furthermore, patients who received greater than 500 PUVA treatments were 19 times more likely to develop SCC. The risk of SCC was not lower 15 years after stopping treatment versus those continuing to receive PUVA treatment. Additionally, patients previously treated with PUVA followed by cyclosporine had an even higher risk of developing skin cancer [57].

A review of more than 13,000 patients undergoing Goeckerman therapy demonstrated no increased risk of cancer with the use of CCT with corticosteroids in psoriasis or AD patients [58]. At the Mayo Clinic, two large 25-year follow-up studies showed no significant increase in the incidence of cancer in AD and psoriasis patients compared to the general population [59, 60].

## Conclusion

Phototherapy is an effective and safe treatment modality for AD in patients who have failed topical treatments. NB-UVB can be used safely in pediatric patients and pregnant or nursing women. NB-UVB is currently the most widely used modality due to lack of systemic side effects and ease of administration. The limitations of in-office phototherapy include local availability, missed work or school, need for reliable transportation, and out-of-pocket costs with some insurances. For select patients, home phototherapy is an option. The most common side effects of phototherapy are erythema, itching, burning, and xerosis. Long-term side effects include tanning and photoaging. While long-term PUVA (>200 treatment sessions) may increase the risk of skin cancer, there is no convincing evidence of an increased risk of skin cancer with UVB phototherapy. Combination therapy such as phototherapy plus topical agents and biologic agents is commonly employed in clinical practice, but long-term randomized clinical trials are needed to better understand its safety and efficacy.

**Board Review Question Explanation**
At this time, what therapy would you recommend to the patient?

A. Trimethoprim–sulfamethoxazole
B. Narrowband ultraviolet B (NB-UVB) phototherapy (correct)
C. Continue current regimen
D. Methotrexate
E. Dilute bleach baths and emollients

**Explanation**
The patient has atopic dermatitis that has failed treatment with topical and oral corticosteroids, topical calcineurin inhibitors, and antihistamines. At this point, a second-line treatment would include phototherapy, which may be used in patients with atopic dermatitis recalcitrant to topical medications. NB-UVB is currently the most widely used form of phototherapy for the treatment of atopic dermatitis and results in approximately half of patients achieving clear or almost clear skin when used in combination with topical corticosteroids [61]. NB-UVB phototherapy is a good option for this patient who is of childbearing potential and considering pregnancy. NB-UVB phototherapy may safely be used in women who are pregnant or breastfeeding, while systemic agents such as methotrexate should be avoided. The side effect profile of phototherapy is favorable in comparison to systemic immunosuppressive agents. The most notable acute side effects of phototherapy include erythema, burning, itching, and xerosis. Long-term side effects include tanning and photoaging. NB-UVB must be administered three times per week for at least 12 weeks to see significant improvement. This patient has a flexible work schedule; therefore, in-office NB-UVB treatments are feasible.

**Key Takeaway Points**

- Phototherapy is an effective and safe treatment option for patients with moderate to severe atopic dermatitis who have failed topical treatments.
- Currently available phototherapy modalities for atopic dermatitis include broadband ultraviolet B (BB-UVB) (290–320 nm), narrowband UVB (311–313 nm), excimer laser (308 nm), psoralen plus ultraviolet A (PUVA), and Goeckerman therapy (UVB plus crude coal tar), although BB-UVB is no longer widely available and Goeckerman is only performed at select centers.

- Ultraviolet B (UVB) phototherapy can be used safely in pediatric, pregnant, and nursing populations.
- The acute side effects of phototherapy include erythema, itching, burning, and xerosis. Long-term side effects of phototherapy include tanning and photoaging. The risk of skin cancer is only increased in White patients who have undergone extensive PUVA therapy (greater than 200 treatment sessions).
- While phototherapy is typically administered in the office setting and requires three times per week treatments initially, there are options for home phototherapy in appropriate situations.

## References


1. Rodenbeck DL, Silverberg JI, Silverberg NB. Phototherapy for atopic dermatitis. Clin Dermatol. 2016;34(5):607–13. https://doi.org/10.1016/j.clindermatol.2016.05.011.
2. Aatrizi A, Raone B, Ravaioli GM. Management of atopic dermatitis: safety and efficacy of phototherapy. Clin Cosmet Investig Dermatol. 2015;8:511–20. Published 2015 Oct 5. https://doi.org/10.2147/CCID.S87987.
3. Morison WL, Parrish J, Fitzpatrick TB. Oral psoralen photochemotherapy of atopic eczema. Br J Dermatol. 1978;98(1):25–30. https://doi.org/10.1111/j.1365-2133.1978.tb07329.x.
4. Tartar D, Bhutani T, Huynh M, Berger T, Koo J. Update on the immunological mechanism of action behind phototherapy. J Drugs Dermatol. 2014;13(5):564–8.
5. el-Ghorr AA, Norval M. Biological effects of narrow-band (311 nm TL01) UVB irradiation: a review. J Photochem Photobiol B. 1997;38(2–3):99–106. https://doi.org/10.1016/s1011-1344(96)07454-4.
6. Schwarz T. The dark and the sunny sides of UVR-induced immunosuppression: photoimmunology revisited. J Invest Dermatol. 2010;130(1):49–54. https://doi.org/10.1038/jid.2009.217.
7. Tay YK, Morelli JG, Weston WL. Experience with UVB phototherapy in children. Pediatr Dermatol. 1996;13(5):406–9. https://doi.org/10.1111/j.1525-1470.1996.tb00711.x.
8. Placek W, Kaszuba A, Lesiak A, et al. Phototherapy and photochemotherapy in dermatology. Recommendations of the Polish Dermatological Society. Dermatol Rev. 2019;106(3):237–56. https://doi.org/10.5114/dr.2019.86906.
9. Rathod DG, Muneer H, Masood S. Phototherapy. In: StatPearls. Treasure Island (FL): StatPearls Publishing; 2022. https://www.ncbi.nlm.nih.gov/books/NBK563140/.
10. Koek MB, Sigurdsson V, van Weelden H, Steegmans PH, Bruijnzeel-Koomen CA, Buskens E. Cost effectiveness of home ultraviolet B phototherapy for psoriasis: economic evaluation of a randomised controlled trial (PLUTO study). BMJ. 2010;340:c1490. Published 2010 Apr 20. https://doi.org/10.1136/bmj.c1490.
11. Sidbury R, Davis DM, Cohen DE, et al. Guidelines of care for the management of atopic dermatitis: section 3. Management and treatment with phototherapy and systemic agents. J Am Acad Dermatol. 2014;71(2):327–49. https://doi.org/10.1016/j.jaad.2014.03.030.
12. Heckman CJ, Chandler R, Kloss JD, et al. Minimal erythema dose (MED) testing. J Vis Exp. 2013;75:e50175. Published 2013 May 28. https://doi.org/10.3791/50175.
13. Grundmann SA, Beissert S. Modern aspects of phototherapy for atopic dermatitis. J Allergy (Cairo). 2012;2012:121797. https://doi.org/10.1155/2012/121797.
14. Pérez-Ferriols A, Aranegui B, Pujol-Montcusí JA, et al. Phototherapy in atopic dermatitis: a systematic review of the literature. Actas Dermosifiliogr. 2015;106(5):387–401. https://doi.org/10.1016/j.ad.2014.12.017.

15. Meduri NB, Vandergriff T, Rasmussen H, Jacobe H. Phototherapy in the management of atopic dermatitis: a systematic review. Photodermatol Photoimmunol Photomed. 2007;23(4):106–12. https://doi.org/10.1111/j.1600-0781.2007.00291.x.
16. Heinlin J, Schiffner-Rohe J, Schiffner R, Einsele-Krämer B, Landthaler M, Klein A, et al. A first prospective randomized controlled trial on the efficacy and safety of synchronous balneophototherapy vs. narrow-band UVB monotherapy for atopic dermatitis. J Eur Acad Dermatol Venereol. 2011;25(7):765–73.
17. Tintle S, Shemer A, Suárez-Fariñas M, et al. Reversal of atopic dermatitis with narrowband UVB phototherapy and biomarkers for therapeutic response. J Allergy Clin Immunol. 2011;128(3):583–93.e934. https://doi.org/10.1016/j.jaci.2011.05.042.
18. Clayton TH, Clark SM, Turner D, Goulden V. The treatment of severe atopic dermatitis in childhood with narrowband ultraviolet B phototherapy. Clin Exp Dermatol. 2007;32(1):28–33. https://doi.org/10.1111/j.1365-2230.2006.02292.
19. Dayal S, Pathak K, Sahu P, Jain VK. Narrowband UV-B phototherapy in childhood atopic dermatitis: efficacy and safety. An Bras Dermatol. 2017;92(6):801–6. https://doi.org/10.1590/abd1806-4841.20175958.
20. Darné S, Leech SN, Taylor AE. Narrowband ultraviolet B phototherapy in children with moderate-to-severe eczema: a comparative cohort study. Br J Dermatol. 2014;170(1):150–6. https://doi.org/10.1111/bjd.12580.
21. Ortiz-Salvador JM, Pérez-Ferriols A. Phototherapy in atopic dermatitis. Adv Exp Med Biol. 2017;996:279–86. https://doi.org/10.1007/978-3-319-56017-5_23.
22. Jekler J, Larkö O. Combined UVA-UVB versus UVB phototherapy for atopic dermatitis: a paired-comparison study. J Am Acad Dermatol. 1990;22(1):49–53. https://doi.org/10.1016/0190-9622(90)70006-4.
23. George SA, Bilsland DJ, Johnson BE, Ferguson J. Narrow-band (TL-01) UVB air-conditioned phototherapy for chronic severe adult atopic dermatitis. Br J Dermatol. 1993;128(1):49–56. https://doi.org/10.1111/j.1365-2133.1993.tb00147.x.
24. Rooney JF, Straus SE, Mannix ML, et al. UV light-induced reactivation of herpes simplex virus type 2 and prevention by acyclovir. J Infect Dis. 1992;166(3):500–6. https://doi.org/10.1093/infdis/166.3.500.
25. Babalola O, Strober BE. Treatment of atopic dermatitis in pregnancy. Dermatol Ther. 2013;26(4):293–301. https://doi.org/10.1111/dth.12074.
26. El-Saie LT, Rabie AR, Kamel MI, Seddeik AK, Elsaie ML. Effect of narrowband ultraviolet B phototherapy on serum folic acid levels in patients with psoriasis. Lasers Med Sci. 2011;26(4):481–5. https://doi.org/10.1007/s10103-011-0895-0.
27. Juzeniene A, Stokke KT, Thune P, Moan J. Pilot study of folate status in healthy volunteers and in patients with psoriasis before and after UV exposure. J Photochem Photobiol B. 2010;101(2):111–6. https://doi.org/10.1016/j.jphotobiol.2010.01.013.
28. Rose RF, Batchelor RJ, Turner D, Goulden V. Narrowband ultraviolet B phototherapy does not influence serum and red cell folate levels in patients with psoriasis. J Am Acad Dermatol. 2009;61(2):259–62. https://doi.org/10.1016/j.jaad.2009.03.011.
29. Zhang M, Goyert G, Lim HW. Folate and phototherapy: what should we inform our patients? J Am Acad Dermatol. 2017;77(5):958–64. https://doi.org/10.1016/j.jaad.2016.10.016.
30. Dennis M, Bhutani T, Koo J, Liao W. Goeckerman therapy for the treatment of eczema: a practical guide and review of efficacy. J Dermatol Treat. 2013;24(1):2–6. https://doi.org/10.3109/09546634.2011.607794.
31. Farahnik B, Beroukhim K, Danesh M, et al. Successful use of a modified Goeckerman regimen in the treatment of chronic severe atopic dermatitis: a prospective pilot study. J Am Acad Dermatol. 2016;75(5):1068–71. https://doi.org/10.1016/j.jaad.2016.06.040.
32. de Miguel R, el-Azhary R. Efficacy, safety, and cost of Goeckerman therapy compared with biologics in the treatment of moderate to severe psoriasis. Int J Dermatol. 2009;48(6):653–8. https://doi.org/10.1111/j.1365-4632.2009.04012.x.

33. Thibodeaux Q, Beck K, Lockshin BN, et al. Treatment of plaque psoriasis with an excimer laser utilizing an optimal therapeutic UVB dose protocol. J Drugs Dermatol. 2020;19(4):49–354. https://doi.org/10.36849/JDD.2020.489.
34. Baltás E, Csoma Z, Bodai L, Ignácz F, Dobozy A, Kemény L. Treatment of atopic dermatitis with the xenon chloride excimer laser. J Eur Acad Dermatol Venereol. 2006;20(6):657–60. https://doi.org/10.1111/j.1468-3083.2006.01495.x.
35. Shroff A, Malajian D, Czarnowicki T, et al. Use of 308 nm excimer laser for the treatment of chronic hand and foot eczema. Int J Dermatol. 2016;55(8):e447–53. https://doi.org/10.1111/ijd.13205.
36. Syed S, Weibel L, Kennedy H, Harper JI. A pilot study showing pulsed-dye laser treatment improves localized areas of chronic atopic dermatitis. Clin Exp Dermatol. 2008;33(3):243–8. https://doi.org/10.1111/j.1365-2230.2007.02644.x.
37. Farahnik B, Nakamura M, Singh RK, et al. The patient's guide to psoriasis treatment. Part 2: PUVA phototherapy. Dermatol Ther (Heidelb). 2016;6(3):315–24. https://doi.org/10.1007/s13555-016-0130-9.
38. Atherton DJ, Carabott F, Glover MT, Hawk JL. The role of psoralen photochemotherapy (PUVA) in the treatment of severe atopic eczema in adolescents. Br J Dermatol. 1988;118(6):791–5. https://doi.org/10.1111/j.1365-2133.1988.tb02597.x.
39. Sheehan MP, Atherton DJ, Norris P, Hawk J. Oral psoralen photochemotherapy in severe childhood atopic eczema: an update. Br J Dermatol. 1993;129(4):431–6. https://doi.org/10.1111/j.1365-2133.1993.tb03171.x.
40. O'Connor OA, Bhagat G, Ganapathi KA, et al. T-cell lymphomas. In: Hematology. Elsevier; 2018. p. 1343–80. https://doi.org/10.1016/b978-0-323-35762-3.00085-8.
41. Musters AH, Mashayekhi S, Harvey J, et al. Phototherapy for atopic eczema. Cochrane Database Syst Rev. 2021;10(10):CD013870. Published 2021 Oct 28. https://doi.org/10.1002/14651858.CD013870.pub2.
42. Thatiparthi A, Martin A, Liu J, Wu JJ. Home phototherapy during the COVID-19 pandemic. Cutis. 2021;107(2):87–8. https://doi.org/10.12788/cutis.0172.
43. Bawany F. Home phototherapy: improving access to dermatologic care. J Am Acad Dermatol. 2022;87(3):AB65.
44. Nolan BV, Yentzer BA, Feldman SR. A review of home phototherapy for psoriasis. Dermatol Online J. 2010;16(2):1.
45. Feldman SR, Clark A, Reboussin DM, Fleischer AB Jr. An assessment of potential problems of home phototherapy treatment of psoriasis. Cutis. 1996;58(1):71–3.
46. Cameron H, Yule S, Dawe RS, Ibbotson SH, Moseley H, Ferguson J. Review of an established UK home phototherapy service 1998–2011: improving access to a cost-effective treatment for chronic skin disease. Public Health. 2014;128(4):317–24.
47. Rajpara AN, O'Neill JL, Nolan BV, Yentzer BA, Feldman SR. Review of home phototherapy. Dermatol Online J. 2010;16(12):2. Published 2010 Dec 15.
48. Tzung TY, Lin CB, Chen YH, Yang CY. Pimecrolimus and narrowband UVB as monotherapy or combination therapy in children and adolescents with atopic dermatitis. Acta Derm Venereol. 2006;86(1):34–8. https://doi.org/10.1080/00015550510044163.
49. Fernández-Guarino M, Aboin-Gonzalez S, Barchino L, Velazquez D, Arsuaga C, Lázaro P. Treatment of moderate and severe adult chronic atopic dermatitis with narrow-band UVB and the combination of narrow-band UVB/UVA phototherapy. Dermatol Ther. 2016;29(1):19–23. https://doi.org/10.1111/dth.12273.
50. Rossi M, Rovati C, Arisi M, et al. A short cycle of narrow-band UVB phototherapy in the early phase of dupilumab therapy can provide a quicker improvement of severe atopic dermatitis. Dermatology. 2021;237(3):407–15. https://doi.org/10.1159/000512456.
51. Gori N, Chiricozzi A, Malvaso D, et al. Successful combination of systemic agents for the treatment of atopic dermatitis resistant to dupilumab therapy. Dermatology. 2021;237(4):535–41. https://doi.org/10.1159/000512890.
52. Ahad T, Wang EY, Liu YA, et al. Incidence of skin cancers in patients with eczema treated with ultraviolet phototherapy. J Am Acad Dermatol. 2022;87(2):387–9. https://doi.org/10.1016/j.jaad.2021.11.048.

53. Hearn RM, Kerr AC, Rahim KF, et. al. Incidence of skin cancers in 3867 patients treated with narrow-band ultraviolet B phototherapy. Br J Dermatol. 2008;159:931–5.
54. Karaosmanoglu N, Ozdemir Cetinkaya P, Kutlu O, et al. A cross-sectional analysis of skin cancer risk in patients receiving narrow-band ultraviolet B phototherapy: an evaluation of 100 patients. Arch Dermatol Res. 2020;312(4):249–53. https://doi.org/10.1007/s00403-019-02007-7.
55. Osmancevic A, Gillstedt M, Wennberg AM, Larkö O. The risk of skin cancer in psoriasis patients treated with UVB therapy. Acta Derm Venereol. 2014;94(4):425–30. https://doi.org/10.2340/00015555-1753.
56. Nijsten TE, Stern RS. The increased risk of skin cancer is persistent after discontinuation of psoralen + ultraviolet A: a cohort study. J Invest Dermatol. 2003;121(2):252–8. https://doi.org/10.1046/j.1523-1747.2003.12350.x.
57. Marcil I, Stern RS. Squamous-cell cancer of the skin in patients given PUVA and cyclosporine: nested cohort crossover study. Lancet. 2001;358(9287):1042–5. https://doi.org/10.1016/S0140-6736(01)06179-7.
58. Roelofzen JH, Aben KK, Oldenhof UT, et al. No increased risk of cancer after coal tar treatment in patients with psoriasis or eczema. J Invest Dermatol. 2010;130(4):953–61. https://doi.org/10.1038/jid.2009.389.
59. Maughan WZ, Muller SA, Perry HO, Pittelkow MR, O'Brien PC. Incidence of skin cancers in patients with atopic dermatitis treated with coal tar. A 25-year follow-up study. J Am Acad Dermatol. 1980;3(6):612–5. https://doi.org/10.1016/s0190-9622(80)80075-2.
60. Pittelkow MR, Perry HO, Muller SA, Maughan WZ, O'Brien PC. Skin cancer in patients with psoriasis treated with coal tar. A 25-year follow-up study. Arch Dermatol. 1981;117(8):465–8.
61. Choi JY, Owusu-Ayim M, Dawe R, Ibbotson S, Fleming C, Foerster J. Narrowband ultraviolet B phototherapy is associated with a reduction in topical corticosteroid and clinical improvement in atopic dermatitis: a historical inception cohort study. Clin Exp Dermatol. 2021;46(6):1067–74. https://doi.org/10.1111/ced.14676.

# Chapter 10
# Treatment of AD with Dupilumab

**Michael Ryan Collier, Brandon Smith, Shivali Devjani, Priya Engel, and Jashin J. Wu**

**Case Title** A 2-year-old male with worsening atopic dermatitis.

**Case**

A 2-year-old male with a history of atopic dermatitis is brought to your clinic by his mother for a follow-up visit. The patient was originally diagnosed at 6 months of age when he presented with erythematous, pruritic papules and vesicles distributed over the face and posterior elbows. He was initially treated with low-potency topical corticosteroids and experienced some improvement, but escalation to higher-potency topical steroids and tacrolimus was required at his most recent visit. Despite these treatments, the rash has continually worsened and progressed to now involve the bilateral face, elbows, knees, and buttocks. He has no other known past medical history, but his mother reports that he has developed new episodic wheezing that has worsened over the past 6 months. She also reports that he has become increasingly irritable and has

---

M. R. Collier
University of South Florida, Morsani College of Medicine, Tampa, FL, USA
e-mail: mrcollier@usf.edu

B. Smith
Drexel University College of Medicine, Philadelphia, PA, USA
e-mail: bs983@drexel.edu

S. Devjani
SUNY Downstate College of Medicine, New York, NY, USA
e-mail: shivali.devjani@downstate.edu

P. Engel
California University of Science and Medicine, Colton, CA, USA
e-mail: vedulap@cusm.org

J. J. Wu (✉)
University of Miami Miller School of Medicine, Miami, FL, USA



N. Brownstone et al. (eds.), *Clinical Cases in Atopic Dermatitis*, Clinical Cases in Dermatology, https://doi.org/10.1007/978-3-031-52147-8_10

difficulty sleeping through the night. Allergen testing completed at a prior visit was unremarkable, and his mother is careful to avoid any irritants that could worsen his condition.

**Board Review Question**
Based on the clinical case description, which of the following is the most appropriate long-term treatment for the patient?

A. Prednisone
B. Calcipotriene
C. Methotrexate
D. Dupilumab
E. Abrocitinib

# Main Text

## *Background*

Dupilumab is a fully human monoclonal antibody that first received FDA approval for the treatment of atopic dermatitis (AD) in 2017. Since then, it has subsequently been approved for the treatment of asthma, chronic rhinosinusitis with nasal polyposis (CRSwNP), and eosinophilic esophagitis as well [1, 2]. The mechanism of action of dupilumab involves inhibiting the activity of interleukin-4 (IL-4) and interleukin-13 (IL-13), both of which are integral components of the type 2 helper T-cell (Th2) immune response [3]. Specifically, dupilumab binds avidly to the shared alpha subunit of the IL-4 receptor, preventing both IL-4 and IL-13 from binding their receptors and activating further downstream signaling. Given the selectivity with which dupilumab inhibits the Th2 response, it is well suited as a treatment for conditions where pathologic activation of the response is a known driver, namely the "atopic triad" of asthma, atopic dermatitis, and chronic rhinosinusitis [4].

While a variety of systemic immunosuppressants have long been used off-label as part of AD management [5], dupilumab was the first systemic therapy, besides corticosteroids, to receive FDA approval for the treatment of AD. As a monoclonal antibody (mAb), it was also the first biologic medication to be approved for this indication. That dupilumab is a fully human mAb, as opposed to murine, chimeric, or partially humanized, is important as it relates to the efficacy and side effect profile of the medication. The latter three types all contain some non-human epitopes that are more likely to elicit host immune responses, which can result in decreased efficacy and increased frequency of adverse events with these treatments [6]. Thus, dupilumab, by virtue of being a fully human mAb that targets the Th2 response selectively, was optimally positioned from the beginning of its development to be an effective and relatively safe systemic therapy for the long-term management of AD.

## *Efficacy*

Results from the first phase 1 randomized controlled trial (RCT) investigating the use of dupilumab for the treatment of AD demonstrated significant reductions in Eczema Area and Severity Index (EASI) and Investigator's Global Assessment (IGA) scores with dupilumab use as compared to placebo [7]. A subsequent phase 2b extension produced similar score reductions with dupilumab doses as low as 100 mg every 4 weeks, though the degree of response was dose-dependent [8]. The initial phase 3 extension consisted of the identical SOLO 1 and SOLO 2 trials, both of which compared dupilumab to placebo among adults with moderate-to-severe AD who had experienced an inadequate response to topical therapies. In these studies, 36–37% of the patients receiving dupilumab 300 mg weekly, 36–38% of those receiving dupilumab 300 mg every other week, and 8–10% of those receiving placebo reached an IGA score of 0 or 1 (indicating clear or almost clear disease) following 16 weeks of treatment [9]. These early results demonstrated the superiority of dupilumab over placebo in achieving a clinically meaningful improvement for patients with AD.

Following the publication of results from the SOLO 1 and SOLO 2 trials, additional studies utilizing RCT-derived data found similar efficacy with dupilumab use among a variety of racial subgroups [10, 11] and among patients who had previously failed other systemic AD therapies [12, 13]. Patients receiving long-term dupilumab were found to have maintained their initial response after 52 weeks of therapy, but those who withdrew from treatment or received dose reductions experienced loss of this response in a dose-dependent manner [14, 15]. Numerous studies also found significant improvement in patient-reported outcomes including anxiety and depression, sleep, and itch with dupilumab use [16–20]. One pooled analysis of phase 3 clinical trials found significant improvement in Peak Pruritus Numerical Rating Scale (NRS) scores as early as treatment day 2 and a mean percent decrease in NRS as high as 57.3% by treatment end [21]. Importantly, multiple clinical trials also demonstrated that dupilumab was similarly effective in treating pediatric AD, with similar improvements in EASI, IGA, and NRS scores reported among adolescents and younger children as seen with adults [22–26].

Because dupilumab was one of the first systemic therapies to be approved for the treatment of moderate-to-severe AD, few clinical trials have directly compared its efficacy to that of other systemic therapies. Exceptions to this can be found with the relatively new Janus kinase (JAK) inhibitors, some of which were studied using dupilumab-treated patients as comparator groups. Abrocitinib and upadacitinib, for example, were both found to produce similar or slightly greater reductions in EASI and IGA scores than dupilumab depending on the dose studied [27–30]. Most meta-analyses that have examined the comparative efficacies of a wide variety of systemic AD treatments have generally found dupilumab, abrocitinib, and upadacitinib to be the most effective treatments [31–36]. Among such studies, dupilumab has generally been found to be superior to conventional immunosuppressants such as cyclosporine, methotrexate, mycophenolate mofetil, and azathioprine in treating AD.

## *Side Effects and Safety*

The first RCTs that investigated dupilumab use among adult and pediatric patients with AD found it to be generally well tolerated and identified conjunctivitis, injection site reactions, nasopharyngitis, and headache as the most commonly reported adverse events [7–9, 22–26]. No additional major adverse events were initially identified following long-term dupilumab treatment [14, 15], and one meta-analysis of clinical trial data found only conjunctivitis (RR 2.64; 95% CI 1.79–3.89), injection site reactions (RR 2.24; 95% CI 1.68–2.99), and headache (RR 1.47; 95% CI 1.05–2.06) to be significantly increased with dupilumab use relative to placebo [37]. A systematic review and meta-analysis that included 3303 AD patients across 22 studies reported pooled incidences of the most common adverse events seen with dupilumab use (Table 10.1).

Subsequent studies have identified additional side effects including paradoxical head and neck erythema, psoriasis, inflammatory arthritis/arthralgia, and alopecia areata with use of dupilumab among AD patients [39]. Facial redness, in particular, was reported in up to 10.6% of dupilumab-treated patients in one US study [38]. While possible, serious adverse events are rare with dupilumab use, as indicated by a meta-analysis of RCT patients that found dupilumab to be associated with a 32% decreased risk of serious AEs compared to placebo [40]. There has also been shown to be no significant difference in rates of study discontinuation due to adverse events between dupilumab- and placebo-treated patients across RCTs [41].

Given the immunomodulatory effects of dupilumab and the predilection toward cutaneous infections exhibited among AD patients, close monitoring for skin and other infections was conducted across most dupilumab clinical trials. Despite these theoretical risks, dupilumab was repeatedly shown across a number of studies to be associated with a decreased risk of all skin infections, decreased risk of eczema herpeticum, and no significant difference in risk of all infections when compared to placebo [42, 43]. The decreased overall risk of cutaneous infections with dupilumab use has been frequently reported as high as 44% [40, 42].

Laboratory safety is of paramount importance when comparing dupilumab to other available systemic AD treatments. With the exception of eosinophilia, no clinically meaningful changes in routine laboratory parameters have been consistently identified with dupilumab use, and routine monitoring of these values during treatment is not required [44–46]. This stands in contrast to the various systemic

**Table 10.1** Pooled incidence of most commonly reported adverse events with dupilumab use among 3303 AD patients [38]

| Adverse event | Incidence in dupilumab-treated patients (%) |
|---|---|
| Conjunctivitis | 26.1 |
| Blepharitis | 9.6 |
| Keratitis | 6.2 |
| HSV infection | 5.8 |
| Headache | 5.5 |
| Injection site reactions | 5.3 |

immunosuppressants used to treat AD, most of which exhibit the potential for toxicity (e.g., renal, hepatic) and do require routine monitoring. Additionally, dupilumab exhibits a more benign side effect profile when compared to JAK inhibitors such as abrocitinib and upadacitinib, both of which carry an official black box warning with regard to infectious and cardiovascular risks, thrombosis, higher all-cause mortality, and carcinogenic potential [47, 48].

## *Clinical Use of Dupilumab to Treat Atopic Dermatitis*

A number of clinical practice guidelines and recommendations have been put forth to help providers incorporate dupilumab appropriately into their AD treatment plan [49–53]. When considering starting a patient on dupilumab, providers should first assess the extent and severity of the patient's disease using validated clinical severity scales such as the Scoring of Atopic Dermatitis (SCORAD) index or the EASI. For mild AD, emphasis should be placed on non-pharmacologic measures and topical treatments, both of which are discussed more extensively in Chaps. 6–8 of this textbook. Systemic therapies, including dupilumab, should be reserved for those patients with moderate-to-severe disease who have experienced little to no improvement following appropriate use of non-pharmacologic and topical interventions.

Before initiating systemic therapy, prescribers should check that patients are properly adhering to topical treatments and avoiding all potential triggers that could be exacerbating their AD. Identification and treatment of any co-occurring infections should also be completed before initiation of systemic treatments. For older children and adults, additional measures such as phototherapy and/or a short course of systemic immunosuppression may be considered prior to starting systemic therapy. However, it is unclear whether a short course of immunosuppressive therapy or initiation of long-term therapy is more favorable at this stage.

Owing to its relatively favorable efficacy and side effect profile when compared to other systemic treatments, dupilumab is often considered as a first-line agent for patients with recalcitrant AD who require long-term maintenance therapy. It is particularly favored for patients suffering from comorbid atopic diseases, as it has been shown to lead to improvement in outcomes related to these conditions when used among AD patients [54, 55]. One study also found dupilumab use to be associated with a decreased incidence of new asthma and CRSwNP diagnoses when used for the treatment of other atopic diseases [40]. Cost is another factor that must be taken into consideration, as dupilumab is one of the more expensive systemic therapies available for the treatment of AD [56, 57]. Some of this cost, however, is offset by the broader savings on healthcare seen with dupilumab use, including decreased rates of all-cause hospitalizations among AD patients [58, 59]. Systemic immunosuppressants (e.g., cyclosporine, methotrexate, mycophenolate mofetil, azathioprine) may be preferable for some patients with whom cost is a significant concern.

Before starting treatment with dupilumab, patients should be counseled regarding their prognosis and expectations for goals of treatment. Between 30 and 40% of dupilumab-treated patients are likely to experience complete or near-complete resolution of their AD, though it may take up to 3 months or more of treatment to fully realize this benefit [9]. Even patients who don't experience this degree of response can still expect significant improvements, with mean reductions in EASI and pruritus NRS scores being reported at 48.9% and 35.2%, respectively, among such patients [20]. Patients should also be counseled on the side effects most likely to be experienced with dupilumab therapy, which includes ocular complications, facial erythema, and injection site reactions, as discussed previously within this chapter.

Determination of adequate response to dupilumab is provider- and patient-specific and should be based primarily on the patient's individual goals of treatment. For patients who are not already receiving topical therapies, the addition of these treatments may lead to improved outcomes compared to dupilumab alone [9]. Additional measures, such as oral antihistamines for pruritus, can also be incorporated into the treatment plan. Patients experiencing inadequate response may also benefit from the addition of phototherapy to the treatment regimen [60]. Escalation to weekly (as opposed to every other week) dosing may also be attempted, although evidence supporting the benefit of this approach is lacking. Finally, while the safety of combination systemic therapy is not fully known, the addition of conventional immunosuppressants may also be considered for patients with severe disease [39].

Across multiple clinical trials, side effects from dupilumab did not result in higher rates of treatment discontinuation compared to placebo [41]. In practice, early identification and treatment of most side effects often eliminates the need for discontinuation. Depending on patient and provider preference, dose reduction (by increasing the time between injections beyond every other week) may be attempted before deciding to discontinue treatment. Discontinuation is appropriate in the event of hypersensitivity reactions (e.g., anaphylaxis), development of severe eosinophilic conditions (e.g., vasculitic rash, worsening pulmonary/neurological symptoms), and parasitic infections that do not respond to anti-helminth treatment. Live vaccines should also be avoided with dupilumab, and, if the patient is already receiving systemic corticosteroids upon dupilumab initiation, abrupt withdrawal of steroids should be avoided [61]. While no evidence has suggested teratogenic potential with dupilumab, some guidelines have recommended that pregnant and breastfeeding women avoid it given that human IgG antibodies such as dupilumab are known to both cross the placenta and enter into breast milk [62].

Dupilumab is administered via subcutaneous injection by use of a pre-filled pen. The recommended initial loading dose for adults aged ≥18 years with AD is 600 milligrams (mg) (given as two separate 300 mg injections at different sites), followed by a maintenance dose of 300 mg every other week thereafter (Q2W) [2]. The recommended dosing for pediatric patients is stratified by body weight (Tables 10.2 and 10.3).

Adults and adolescents ≥12 years of age with two or more concurrent atopic diseases are recommended to receive the 600 mg loading/300 mg Q2W maintenance dosing schedule. Pediatric patients <12 years of age suffering from two or more of these diseases should follow the pediatric dosing schedules in the tables above.

**Table 10.2** Pediatric dosing of dupilumab for patients aged 6 months to 5 years, stratified by body weight [2, 61]

| Body weight | Initial and subsequent dosage |
|---|---|
| 5 to less than 15 kg | 200 mg (one 200 mg injection) Q4W |
| 15 to less than 30 kg | 300 mg (one 300 mg injection) Q4W |

*kg* kilogram, *mg* milligram, *Q4W* once every 4 weeks

**Table 10.3** Pediatric dosing of dupilumab for patients aged 6–17 years, stratified by body weight [2]

| Body weight | Initial loading dose | Subsequent dosage |
|---|---|---|
| 15 to less than 30 kg | 600 mg (two 300 mg injections) | 300 mg Q4W |
| 30 to less than 60 kg | 400 mg (two 200 mg injections) | 200 mg Q2W |
| 60 kg or more | 600 mg (two 300 mg injections) | 300 mg Q2W |

*kg* kilogram, *mg* milligram, *Q4W* once every 4 weeks, *Q2W* once every other week

**Board Review Question Explanation**

Based on the clinical case description, which of the following is the most appropriate long-term treatment for the patient?

A. Prednisone
B. Calcipotriene
C. Methotrexate
D. Dupilumab (correct)
E. Abrocitinib

**Explanation**

A. Prednisone is a systemic corticosteroid that is administered orally. While it could be considered for the treatment of an acute flare of atopic dermatitis, it is generally avoided in pediatric patients and would be inappropriate for long-term therapy [50].
B. Calcipotriene is a topical vitamin D derivative that is used in the treatment of psoriasis, not atopic dermatitis.
C. Methotrexate is among the systemic immunosuppressants that can be used off-label for maintenance therapy of atopic dermatitis. However, it has a less favorable side effect profile than dupilumab and would not be preferred in pediatric patients [50].
D. **Dupilumab** is a monoclonal antibody that has been FDA approved for patients 6 months and older with moderate-to-severe atopic dermatitis that have not responded to topical therapies. It is the most appropriate long-term treatment for this patient, particularly given his new-onset wheezing (which likely indicates undiagnosed asthma) [1, 2].
E. Abrocitinib is an oral Janus kinase (JAK) inhibitor that is equally effective as dupilumab in treating moderate-to-severe atopic dermatitis. However, due to the potential for more serious side effects, it is generally reserved for patients who have failed other systemic therapies, and it is also not approved for use in pediatric patients [47].

**Key Takeaway Points**

- Dupilumab is a monoclonal antibody that was the first systemic biologic therapy to receive FDA approval for the treatment of atopic dermatitis.
- It works by inhibiting the activity of the cytokines IL-4 and IL-13 at their receptors, blunting the Th2 immune response.
- It is indicated for patients with moderate-to-severe atopic dermatitis ≥6 months of age who have not responded to conventional topical therapies.
- Among systemic treatments for atopic dermatitis, dupilumab exhibits a favorable efficacy and side effect profile and is generally considered to be a first-line agent.
- Patients suffering from comorbid asthma, chronic rhinosinusitis with nasal polyposis, or eosinophilic esophagitis, in addition to atopic dermatitis, should be considered ideal candidates for dupilumab therapy.

**Conflicts of Interest** Dr. Wu is or has been an investigator, consultant, or speaker for AbbVie, Almirall, Amgen, Arcutis, Aristea Therapeutics, Bausch Health, Boehringer Ingelheim, Bristol-Myers Squibb, Dermavant, DermTech, Dr. Reddy's Laboratories, Eli Lilly, EPI Health, Galderma, Janssen, LEO Pharma, Mindera, Novartis, Pfizer, Regeneron, Samsung Bioepis, Sanofi Genzyme, Solius, Sun Pharmaceutical, UCB, and Zerigo Health. Authors Collier, Smith, Devjani, and Engel have no conflicts of interest to declare.

## References

1. Pagan AD, David E, Ungar B, Ghalili S, He H, Guttman-Yassky E. Dupilumab improves clinical scores in children and adolescents with moderate to severe atopic dermatitis: a real-world, single-center study. J Allergy Clin Immunol Pract. 2022;10(9):2378–85.
2. Cather J, Young M, DiRuggiero DC, Tofte S, Williams L, Gonzalez T. A review of phase 3 trials of dupilumab for the treatment of atopic dermatitis in adults, adolescents, and children aged 6 and up. Dermatol Ther (Heidelb). 2022;12(9):2013–38.
3. Wenzel S, Ford L, Pearlman D, Spector S, Sher L, Skobieranda F, et al. Dupilumab in persistent asthma with elevated eosinophil levels. N Engl J Med. 2013;368(26):2455–66.
4. Bachert C, Han JK, Desrosiers M, Hellings PW, Amin N, Lee SE, et al. Efficacy and safety of dupilumab in patients with severe chronic rhinosinusitis with nasal polyps (LIBERTY NP SINUS-24 and LIBERTY NP SINUS-52): results from two multicentre, randomised, double-blind, placebo-controlled, parallel-group phase 3 trials. Lancet. 2019;394(10209):1638–50.
5. Sidbury R, Davis DM, Cohen DE, Cordoro KM, Berger TG, Bergman JN, et al. Guidelines of care for the management of atopic dermatitis: section 3. Management and treatment with phototherapy and systemic agents. J Am Acad Dermatol. 2014;71(2):327–49.
6. Newsome BW, Ernstoff MS. The clinical pharmacology of therapeutic monoclonal antibodies in the treatment of malignancy; have the magic bullets arrived? Br J Clin Pharmacol. 2008;66(1):6–19.
7. Beck LA, Thaçi D, Hamilton JD, Graham NM, Bieber T, Rocklin R, et al. Dupilumab treatment in adults with moderate-to-severe atopic dermatitis. N Engl J Med. 2014;371(2):130–9.
8. Thaçi D, Simpson EL, Beck LA, Bieber T, Blauvelt A, Papp K, et al. Efficacy and safety of dupilumab in adults with moderate-to-severe atopic dermatitis inadequately controlled by topical treatments: a randomised, placebo-controlled, dose-ranging phase 2b trial. Lancet. 2016;387(10013):40–52.

9. Simpson EL, Bieber T, Guttman-Yassky E, Beck LA, Blauvelt A, Cork MJ, et al. Two phase 3 trials of dupilumab versus placebo in atopic dermatitis. N Engl J Med. 2016;375(24):2335–48.
10. Alexis AF, Rendon M, Silverberg JI, Pariser DM, Lockshin B, Griffiths CE, et al. Efficacy of dupilumab in different racial subgroups of adults with moderate-to-severe atopic dermatitis in three randomized, placebo-controlled phase 3 trials. J Drugs Dermatol. 2019;18(8):804–13.
11. Zhao Y, Wu L, Lu Q, Gao X, Zhu X, Yao X, et al. The efficacy and safety of dupilumab in Chinese patients with moderate-to-severe atopic dermatitis: a randomized, double-blind, placebo-controlled study. Br J Dermatol. 2022;186(4):633–41.
12. Simpson EL, Bieber T, Eckert L, Wu R, Ardeleanu M, Graham NM, et al. Patient burden of moderate to severe atopic dermatitis (AD): insights from a phase 2b clinical trial of dupilumab in adults. J Am Acad Dermatol. 2016;74(3):491–8.
13. de Bruin-Weller M, Thaçi D, Smith CH, Reich K, Cork MJ, Radin A, et al. Dupilumab with concomitant topical corticosteroid treatment in adults with atopic dermatitis with an inadequate response or intolerance to ciclosporin A or when this treatment is medically inadvisable: a placebo-controlled, randomized phase III clinical trial (LIBERTY AD CAFÉ). Br J Dermatol. 2018;178(5):1083–101.
14. Blauvelt A, de Bruin-Weller M, Gooderham M, Cather JC, Weisman J, Pariser D, et al. Long-term management of moderate-to-severe atopic dermatitis with dupilumab and concomitant topical corticosteroids (LIBERTY AD CHRONOS): a 1-year, randomised, double-blinded, placebo-controlled, phase 3 trial. Lancet. 2017;389(10086):2287–303.
15. Worm M, Simpson EL, Thaçi D, Bissonnette R, Lacour JP, Beissert S, et al. Efficacy and safety of multiple dupilumab dose regimens after initial successful treatment in patients with atopic dermatitis: a randomized clinical trial. JAMA Dermatol. 2020;156(2):131–43.
16. Simpson EL, Gadkari A, Worm M, Soong W, Blauvelt A, Eckert L, et al. Dupilumab therapy provides clinically meaningful improvement in patient-reported outcomes (PROs): a phase IIb, randomized, placebo-controlled, clinical trial in adult patients with moderate to severe atopic dermatitis (AD). J Am Acad Dermatol. 2016;75(3):506–15.
17. Tsianakas A, Luger TA, Radin A. Dupilumab treatment improves quality of life in adult patients with moderate-to-severe atopic dermatitis: results from a randomized, placebo-controlled clinical trial. Br J Dermatol. 2018;178(2):406–14.
18. Lake E. JAAD Game Changers: dupilumab therapy provides clinically meaningful improvement in patient-reported outcomes (PROs): a phase IIb, randomized, placebo-controlled, clinical trial in adult patients with moderate to severe atopic dermatitis (AD). J Am Acad Dermatol. 2019;80(4):882.
19. Cork MJ, Eckert L, Simpson EL, Armstrong A, Barbarot S, Puig L, et al. Dupilumab improves patient-reported symptoms of atopic dermatitis, symptoms of anxiety and depression, and health-related quality of life in moderate-to-severe atopic dermatitis: analysis of pooled data from the randomized trials SOLO 1 and SOLO 2. J Dermatol Treat. 2020;31(6):606–14.
20. Silverberg JI, Simpson EL, Ardeleanu M, Thaçi D, Barbarot S, Bagel J, et al. Dupilumab provides important clinical benefits to patients with atopic dermatitis who do not achieve clear or almost clear skin according to the Investigator's Global Assessment: a pooled analysis of data from two phase III trials. Br J Dermatol. 2019;181(1):80–7.
21. Silverberg JI, Yosipovitch G, Simpson EL, Kim BS, Wu JJ, Eckert L, et al. Dupilumab treatment results in early and sustained improvements in itch in adolescents and adults with moderate to severe atopic dermatitis: analysis of the randomized phase 3 studies SOLO 1 and SOLO 2, AD ADOL, and CHRONOS. J Am Acad Dermatol. 2020;82(6):1328–36.
22. Simpson EL, Paller AS, Siegfried EC, Boguniewicz M, Sher L, Gooderham MJ, et al. Efficacy and safety of dupilumab in adolescents with uncontrolled moderate to severe atopic dermatitis: a phase 3 randomized clinical trial. JAMA Dermatol. 2020;156(1):44–56.
23. Paller AS, Siegfried EC, Thaçi D, Wollenberg A, Cork MJ, Arkwright PD, et al. Efficacy and safety of dupilumab with concomitant topical corticosteroids in children 6–11 years old with severe atopic dermatitis: a randomized, double-blinded, placebo-controlled phase 3 trial. J Am Acad Dermatol. 2020;83(5):1282–93.

24. Paller AS, Bansal A, Simpson EL, Boguniewicz M, Blauvelt A, Siegfried EC, et al. Clinically meaningful responses to dupilumab in adolescents with uncontrolled moderate-to-severe atopic dermatitis: post-hoc analyses from a randomized clinical trial. Am J Clin Dermatol. 2020;21(1):119–31.
25. Cork MJ, Thaçi D, Eichenfield LF, Arkwright PD, Sun X, Chen Z, et al. Dupilumab provides favourable long-term safety and efficacy in children aged ≥6 to <12 years with uncontrolled severe atopic dermatitis: results from an open-label phase IIa study and subsequent phase III open-label extension study. Br J Dermatol. 2021;184(5):857–70.
26. Paller AS, Siegfried EC, Simpson EL, Cork MJ, Lockshin B, Kosloski MP, et al. A phase 2, open-label study of single-dose dupilumab in children aged 6 months to <6 years with severe uncontrolled atopic dermatitis: pharmacokinetics, safety and efficacy. J Eur Acad Dermatol Venereol. 2021;35(2):464–75.
27. Bieber T, Simpson EL, Silverberg JI, Thaçi D, Paul C, Pink AE, et al. Abrocitinib versus placebo or dupilumab for atopic dermatitis. N Engl J Med. 2021;384(12):1101–12.
28. Reich K, Thyssen JP, Blauvelt A, Eyerich K, Soong W, Rice ZP, et al. Efficacy and safety of abrocitinib versus dupilumab in adults with moderate-to-severe atopic dermatitis: a randomised, double-blind, multicentre phase 3 trial. Lancet. 2022;400(10348):273–82.
29. Eichenfield LF, Flohr C, Sidbury R, Siegfried E, Szalai Z, Galus R, et al. Efficacy and safety of abrocitinib in combination with topical therapy in adolescents with moderate-to-severe atopic dermatitis: the JADE TEEN randomized clinical trial. JAMA Dermatol. 2021;157(10):1165–73.
30. Blauvelt A, Teixeira HD, Simpson EL, Costanzo A, De Bruin-Weller M, Barbarot S, et al. Efficacy and safety of upadacitinib vs dupilumab in adults with moderate-to-severe atopic dermatitis: a randomized clinical trial. JAMA Dermatol. 2021;157(9):1047–55.
31. Snast I, Reiter O, Hodak E, Friedland R, Mimouni D, Leshem YA. Are biologics efficacious in atopic dermatitis? A systematic review and meta-analysis. Am J Clin Dermatol. 2018;19(2):145–65.
32. Drucker AM, Ellis AG, Bohdanowicz M, Mashayekhi S, Yiu ZZN, Rochwerg B, et al. Systemic immunomodulatory treatments for patients with atopic dermatitis: a systematic review and network meta-analysis. JAMA Dermatol. 2020;156(6):659–67.
33. Silverberg JI, Thyssen JP, Fahrbach K, Mickle K, Cappelleri JC, Romero W, et al. Comparative efficacy and safety of systemic therapies used in moderate-to-severe atopic dermatitis: a systematic literature review and network meta-analysis. J Eur Acad Dermatol Venereol. 2021;35(9):1797–810.
34. Siegels D, Heratizadeh A, Abraham S, Binnmyr J, Brockow K, Irvine AD, et al. Systemic treatments in the management of atopic dermatitis: a systematic review and meta-analysis. Allergy. 2021;76(4):1053–76.
35. Drucker AM, Morra DE, Prieto-Merino D, Ellis AG, Yiu ZZN, Rochwerg B, et al. Systemic immunomodulatory treatments for atopic dermatitis: update of a living systematic review and network meta-analysis. JAMA Dermatol. 2022;158(5):523–32.
36. Tan XL, Thomas BR, Tan YJ, O'Toole EA. Effects of systemic therapies on pruritus in adults with atopic dermatitis: a systematic review and meta-analysis. Clin Exp Dermatol. 2022;47(4):658–66.
37. Ou Z, Chen C, Chen A, Yang Y, Zhou W. Adverse events of dupilumab in adults with moderate-to-severe atopic dermatitis: a meta-analysis. Int Immunopharmacol. 2018;54:303–10.
38. Halling AS, Loft N, Silverberg JI, Guttman-Yassky E, Thyssen JP. Real-world evidence of dupilumab efficacy and risk of adverse events: a systematic review and meta-analysis. J Am Acad Dermatol. 2021;84(1):139–47.
39. Narla S, Silverberg JI, Simpson EL. Management of inadequate response and adverse effects to dupilumab in atopic dermatitis. J Am Acad Dermatol. 2022;86(3):628–36.
40. Chen X, Liu M, Wu S, Huang Z, Li X, Lai X, et al. Treatment-emergent adverse events in dupilumab-treated patients with allergic diseases: a meta-analysis. Allergy. 2021;76(2):593–6.

41. Han Y, Chen Y, Liu X, Zhang J, Su H, Wen H, et al. Efficacy and safety of dupilumab for the treatment of adult atopic dermatitis: a meta-analysis of randomized clinical trials. J Allergy Clin Immunol. 2017;140(3):888–891.e6.
42. Fleming P, Drucker AM. Risk of infection in patients with atopic dermatitis treated with dupilumab: a meta-analysis of randomized controlled trials. J Am Acad Dermatol. 2018;78(1):62–69.e1.
43. Paller AS, Beck LA, Blauvelt A, Siegfried EC, Cork MJ, Wollenberg A, et al. Infections in children and adolescents treated with dupilumab in pediatric clinical trials for atopic dermatitis—a pooled analysis of trial data. Pediatr Dermatol. 2022;39(2):187–96.
44. Wollenberg A, Beck LA, Blauvelt A, Simpson EL, Chen Z, Chen Q, et al. Laboratory safety of dupilumab in moderate-to-severe atopic dermatitis: results from three phase III trials (LIBERTY AD SOLO 1, LIBERTY AD SOLO 2, LIBERTY AD CHRONOS). Br J Dermatol. 2020;182(5):1120–35.
45. Siegfried EC, Bieber T, Simpson EL, Paller AS, Beck LA, Boguniewicz M, et al. Effect of dupilumab on laboratory parameters in adolescents with atopic dermatitis: results from a randomized, placebo-controlled, phase 3 clinical trial. Am J Clin Dermatol. 2021;22(2):243–55.
46. Paller AS, Wollenberg A, Siegfried E, Thaçi D, Cork MJ, Arkwright PD, et al. Laboratory safety of dupilumab in patients aged 6–11 years with severe atopic dermatitis: results from a phase III clinical trial. Paediatr Drugs. 2021;23(5):515–27.
47. Pfizer Inc. Cibinqo (abrocitinib) [package insert]. U.S. Food and Drug Administration website. https://www.accessdata.fda.gov/drugsatfda_docs/label/2022/213871s000lbl.pdf. Approved January 2022. Accessed 22 July 2022.
48. AbbVie, Inc. Rinvoq (upadacitinib) [package insert]. U.S. Food and Drug Administration website. https://www.accessdata.fda.gov/drugsatfda_docs/label/2022/211675s003lbl.pdf. Revised April 2022. Accessed 22 July 2022.
49. Wollenberg A, Barbarot S, Bieber T, Christen-Zaech S, Deleuran M, Fink-Wagner A, et al. Consensus-based European guidelines for treatment of atopic eczema (atopic dermatitis) in adults and children: part I. J Eur Acad Dermatol Venereol. 2018;32(5):657–82.
50. Wollenberg A, Barbarot S, Bieber T, Christen-Zaech S, Deleuran M, Fink-Wagner A, et al. Consensus-based European guidelines for treatment of atopic eczema (atopic dermatitis) in adults and children: part II. J Eur Acad Dermatol Venereol. 2018;32(6):850–78.
51. Thyssen JP, Berents T, Bradley M, Deleuran M, Grimstad Ø, Korhonen L, et al. Clinical management of atopic dermatitis in adults: mapping of expert opinion in 4 Nordic countries using a modified Delphi process. Acta Derm Venereol. 2020;100(1):adv00015.
52. Smith S, Baker C, Gebauer K, Rubel D, Frankum B, Soyer HP, et al. Atopic dermatitis in adults: an Australian management consensus. Australas J Dermatol. 2020;61(1):23–32.
53. Ghazal S, Ridha Z, D'Aguanno K, Nassim D, Quaiattini A, Netchiporouk E, et al. Treatment guidelines for atopic dermatitis since the approval of dupilumab: a systematic review and quality appraisal using AGREE-II. Front Med (Lausanne). 2022;9:821871.
54. Boguniewicz M, Beck LA, Sher L, Guttman-Yassky E, Thaçi D, Blauvelt A, et al. Dupilumab improves asthma and sinonasal outcomes in adults with moderate to severe atopic dermatitis. J Allergy Clin Immunol Pract. 2021;9(3):1212–1223.e6.
55. Canonica GW, Bourdin A, Peters AT, Desrosiers M, Bachert C, Weidinger S, et al. Dupilumab demonstrates rapid onset of response across three type 2 inflammatory diseases. J Allergy Clin Immunol Pract. 2022;10(6):1515–26.
56. Eichenfield LF, DiBonaventura M, Xenakis J, Lafeuille MH, Duh MS, Fakih I, et al. Costs and treatment patterns among patients with atopic dermatitis using advanced therapies in the United States: analysis of a retrospective claims database. Dermatol Ther (Heidelb). 2020;10(4):791–806.
57. Zimmermann M, Rind D, Chapman R, Kumar V, Kahn S, Carlson J. Economic evaluation of dupilumab for moderate-to-severe atopic dermatitis: a cost-utility analysis. J Drugs Dermatol. 2018;17(7):750–6.

58. Edwards HA, McMeniman EK. The cost of dupilumab treatment for severe atopic dermatitis is largely offset by broader health-care savings and improvement in quality of life. Australas J Dermatol. 2020;61(2):e273–5.
59. Silverberg JI, Rubini NPM, Pires MC, Rossi AB, Zhang A, Chen Z, et al. Dupilumab treatment reduces hospitalizations in adults with moderate-to-severe atopic dermatitis. J Allergy Clin Immunol Pract. 2022;10(5):1279–1285.e1.
60. Rossi M, Rovati C, Arisi M, Tomasi C, Calzavara-Pinton I, Venturini M, et al. A short cycle of narrow-band UVB phototherapy in the early phase of dupilumab therapy can provide a quicker improvement of severe atopic dermatitis. Dermatology. 2021;237(3):407–15.
61. Regeneron Pharmaceuticals, Inc. Dupixent (dupilumab) [package insert]. U.S. Food and Drug Administration website. https://www.accessdata.fda.gov/drugsatfda_docs/label/2022/761055s042lbl.pdf. Revised June 2022. Accessed 20 July 2022.
62. Vestergaard C, Wollenberg A, Thyssen JP. European task force on atopic dermatitis (ETFAD) position paper: treatment of parental atopic dermatitis during preconception, pregnancy and lactation period. J Eur Acad Dermatol Venereol. 2020;34(2):426–7.

# Chapter 11
# Ocular Comorbidities of Atopic Conjunctivitis and Management of Conjunctivitis on Dupilumab Treatment

**Minh T. Nguyen and Gerami D. Seitzman**

**Case Title** A 40-year-old male with red and itchy eyes.

**Case**
It is springtime, and the next patient is a 40-year-old male with asthma, atopic dermatitis, and seasonal allergies who is referred for itchy eyes. As you sit near him and listen to his history of present illness, you note he is rubbing his eyes as he talks. He reports his eyes are intermittently red and itch year-round, though he describes the ocular itching intensifies during the springtime. He does not wear glasses or contact lenses. His vision is not affected. You diagnose him with allergic conjunctivitis in the setting of underlying atopic disease.

**Board Review Question**
Which findings increase the likelihood of dupilumab-induced conjunctivitis?

A. Asthma in addition to dermatitis
B. History of conjunctivitis and more severe baseline dermatitis
C. Chronic eye rubbing behavior
D. Steroid-dependent atopic dermatitis
E. History of contact lens use

M. T. Nguyen · G. D. Seitzman (✉)
Francis I. Proctor Foundation, University of California San Francisco,
San Francisco, CA, USA

Department of Ophthalmology, University of California San Francisco,
San Francisco, CA, USA
e-mail: minh.nguyen3@ucsf.edu; gerami.seitzman@ucsf.edu



N. Brownstone et al. (eds.), *Clinical Cases in Atopic Dermatitis*, Clinical Cases in Dermatology, https://doi.org/10.1007/978-3-031-52147-8_11

## Main Text

### *How Do You Differentiate Allergic Eye Disease from Atopic Eye Disease?*

Allergic conjunctivitis is an IgE-mediated process with seasonal allergic conjunctivitis typically caused by airborne allergens and flaring in spring and summer months. Atopic conjunctivitis is conjunctival inflammation associated with systemic atopy. This inflammatory process occurs year-round and involves both type I and type IV hypersensitivity responses. Allergic conjunctivitis can also compound atopic conjunctivitis. Allergic conjunctivitis typically just involves the conjunctiva, whereas atopic conjunctivitis can involve the conjunctiva and eyelids but may progress to include visually threatening complications such as corneal scarring, cataract, and retinal detachment.

With both allergic and atopic conjunctivitis, ocular findings include eye redness, conjunctival swelling, and marked itching, With atopic conjunctivitis the eyelids typically also demonstrate varying degrees of eczematous dermatitis including skin thickening and excoriation. Eyelids can be thickened and excoriated. Blepharitis, especially staphylococcal blepharitis, is more common with atopic disease [1]. Here the eyelids are red and crusty. With conjunctival involvement, the conjunctival vessels become engorged, and the eye appears hyperemic. The conjunctiva can also become chemotic (swollen and edematous). Visualized using slit lamp microscopy, the conjunctiva becomes inflamed in a characteristic pattern called papillary conjunctivitis (Fig. 11.1). Papillae are conjunctival bumps that form around central blood vessels. Fibrous septae surround the papillae and help form its shape. Small papillae require a slit lamp for identification. Fluorescein dye can pool in the septae and assist with papillae visualization. When atopic eye disease progresses to include the cornea, it is called atopic keratoconjunctivitis (AKC). Early on, the corneal epithelium can be mildly disrupted, noted as punctate corneal epithelial erosions. As this progresses, a larger corneal epithelial defect can develop. If this becomes superinfected into a corneal ulcer, vision loss can occur. Corneal

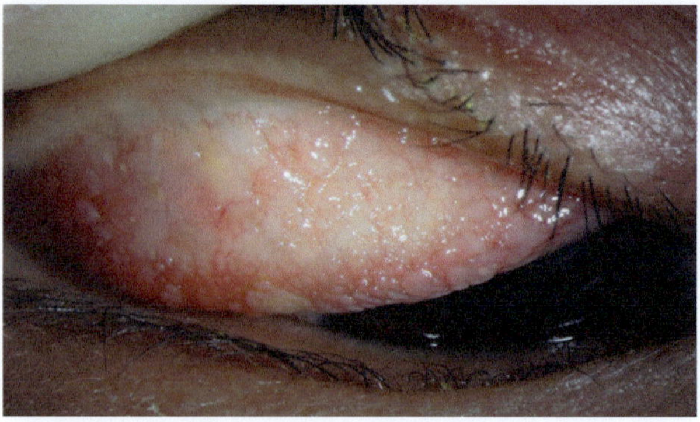

**Fig. 11.1** Severe papillary conjunctivitis. This is an inverted eyelid (flipped inside out). Large papillae (focal inflamed conjunctival elevations) are seen in atopic conjunctivitis

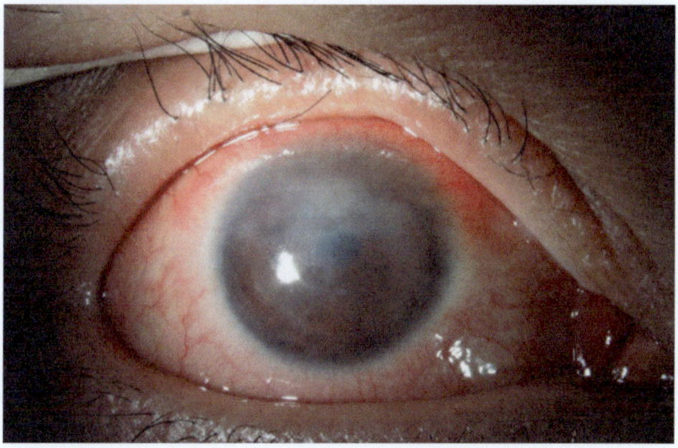

**Fig. 11.2** Atopic keratoconjunctivitis: Severe atopic ocular disease can involve the cornea with corneal neovascularization and visually significant corneal scarring

neovascularization is common in AKC and can lead to visually significant scarring (Fig. 11.2). Herpetic eye disease, especially bilateral herpetic eye disease, is more common with atopy [2].

Severe ocular itching leading to prolonged eye rubbing is common in atopic eye disease.

Rubbing often becomes an unconscious habit, with the frequency of occurrence underestimated by the patient. The repetitive forces of chronic and prolonged eye rubbing can induce many visually significant anatomic structural changes in the eye [3]. Chronic eye rubbing is associated with a corneal thinning disorder called keratoconus [4]. The distortive forces of eye rubbing can be severe enough to cause cataract (clouding of the intraocular lens) and retinal detachments.

## *What Treatment Recommendations Are Appropriate at this Time to Help this Patient with His Itchy Eyes?*

The goals of treatment are to minimize symptoms, prevent flares of disease, and specifically decrease itching so that the urge to rub the eyes is lessened. At this point, our patient does not have any vision complaints and does not have any high-risk eye history such as recent trauma, surgery, or contact lens wear. Mild atopic conjunctivitis is treated like allergic conjunctivitis with a focus on cool compresses and topical mast cell stabilizers. Critical to any therapeutic regimen that requires fingers near eyes is excellent hand hygiene. Cool compresses can promote vasoconstriction. Artificial tears, especially refrigerated, can dilute allergens and inflammatory modulators on the ocular surface. Artificial tear products with a "get the red out" (examples include naphazoline, tetrahydrozoline, oxymetazoline, and brimonidine tartrate) are discouraged as they can result in rebound hyperemia. Topical mast cell stabilizers (examples include olopatadine and ketotifen fumarate) are commonly used and, unless a concomitant preservative allergy is present, can be used chronically without concern for side effects. Preservative-free topical antihistamines and artificial tears are available and should be considered for those with suspected irritation to topical preservatives. With AKC, it is common that over-the-counter regimens are insufficient for symptom control. More potent topical anti-inflammatory therapy is indicated and can be guided by ophthalmologic evaluation.

## *What If the Patient Mentions He Will Start Dupilumab for His Systemic Atopic Disease? What Will You Counsel Him with Regard to His Eyes?*

When used for the indication of atopic dermatitis, 8–22% of patients in clinical trials testing dupilumab developed conjunctivitis [5, 6]. Risk factors for the development of conjunctivitis are prior history of conjunctivitis and more severe baseline systemic dermatitis. Curiously, when used for the indication of asthma, the incidence of conjunctivitis in the dupilumab study group was low and similar to the placebo group [7, 8]. This suggests that dupilumab incites a different mechanism for conjunctivitis in patient with atopic dermatitis than in patients with only asthma. For those who ultimately develop ocular surface inflammation, there does not appear to be an effective way of preventing conjunctivitis. The conjunctivitis that develops can range from mild to severe. Treatment varies depending on conjunctivitis severity [9].

With mild atopic conjunctivitis, recommendations are similar to allergic conjunctivitis: topical antihistamines, bland artificial tear solutions, and cool compresses. Though randomized clinical trials demonstrating efficacy are lacking, topical steroid-sparing medications such as cyclosporine and topical tacrolimus can be trialed [10]. As conjunctivitis progresses, ophthalmic preparations of topical corticosteroids are likely required to control ocular surface inflammation. Topical corticosteroids are supplied in various strengths and potencies, and treatment goals should be to find the lowest potency and lowest frequency that allows for ocular surface inflammatory control. Topical steroid-sparing medication can be used to try to limit the frequency of topical corticosteroids. All patients on chronic topical steroid therapy require baseline glaucoma screening risk assessments and regular follow-up from an eye team comfortable in screening for and managing topical steroid ocular side effects.

## *What If, Instead, on Presentation the Patient Describes Decreased Vision and Photophobia, How Are Your Recommendations Altered?*

In short, this patient now requires an urgent visit to ophthalmology. Any patient with atopic disease and acute eye pain and vision changes warrants urgent evaluation. With severe vision loss, or if the patient wears contact lenses and has acute vision loss and eye pain, the visit becomes emergent. Blurry vision and photophobia are common symptoms of acute AKC. Patients with AKC are more likely to have both inflammatory keratitis and secondary infectious keratitis. Any form of progressive keratitis can be vision threatening without careful ophthalmic evaluation and treatment [11]. A large population-based, case-control study shows atopic patients have an increased risk of both herpes simplex and herpes zoster ophthalmicus [2].

In addition to corneal involvement, poorly controlled atopic disease may lead to other visual complications such as retinal detachment, keratoconus, and cataract. Non-intentional self-induced globe trauma from vigorous eye rubbing plays a major role in the development of these conditions. Patient with atopic disease not only have a greater incidence of retinal detachment but also a higher likelihood of severe (larger) retinal detachments and bilateral retinal detachments [12, 13]. Patients with atopy and eye rubbing are more likely to develop keratoconus, a progressive condition of corneal thinning, budging, and scarring [14]. Cataract development is associated with atopic disease (Fig. 11.3) and eye rubbing and can also occur as a side effect of chronic corticosteroid treatment. Though cataracts can now be replaced with cutting-edge intraocular lens technology, prior to ocular surgery, eye rubbing behavior and eyelid and corneal atopic disease must be well controlled.

In addition to acute vision complaints, any patient on chronic recurrent steroid therapy, systemic and topical, should be monitored regularly by an eye care team comfortable with screening for and managing steroid-induced eye complications [15]. Any patient with chronic recurrent atopic keratoconjunctivitis should be monitored closely and regularly with ophthalmology.

## *What If He Started Dupilumab 6 Weeks Ago and Is Noting His Eye Symptoms Are Becoming Progressively Worse with Each Dupixent Injection?*

It is common for patients with atopic dermatitis to have some degree of atopic conjunctivitis at baseline. However, the timing of worsening in this patient suggests for dupilumab-induced conjunctivitis. As demonstrated in dupilumab clinical trials [5, 6],

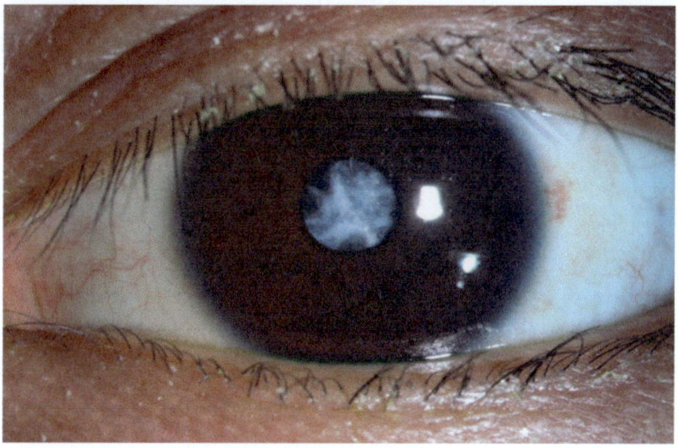

**Fig. 11.3** Anterior subcapsular cataract. Cataracts (clouding of the native intraocular lens) are more frequent in patients with atopic dermatitis

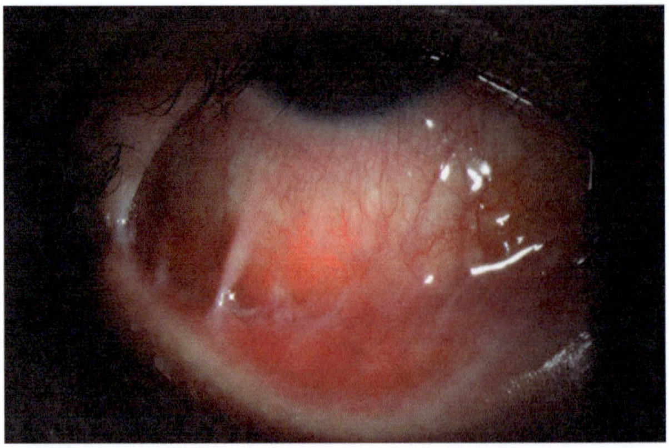

**Fig. 11.4** Severe dupilumab cicatricial conjunctivitis. Dupilumab-induced conjunctivitis ranges from mild to severe. Here, bands of inflamed conjunctival cicatrix connect the lower eyelid to the globe. When cicatricial conjunctivitis develops, drug cessation is commonly recommended

many patients develop conjunctivitis when taking dupilumab. This can develop without a history of conjunctivitis but is more likely to develop with a prior history of conjunctivitis. Also interesting is that conjunctivitis can worsen even when the systemic disease is responding nicely to dupilumab [16]. Dupilumab can induce increasing degrees of conjunctival hyperemia. When the conjunctival injection becomes moderate or severe, commonly the limbus (the conjunctiva that surrounds the cornea) may become relatively more hyperemic and edematous [17]. When very severe, dupilumab can induce an inflammatory cicatricial conjunctivitis (Fig. 11.4), clinically resembling ocular cicatricial pemphigoid [18, 19]. Increased rates of blepharitis (eyelid inflammation) and corneal epithelial keratitis have also been reported [9, 17]. Physicians who prescribe dupilumab should be adept in inquiring about ocular symptoms such as eye irritation, photophobia, pruritus, redness, and discharge. Any patient complaining of vision loss or severe secondary ocular symptoms should be evaluated urgently by ophthalmology.

Similar to treatment of atopic conjunctivitis, treatment for dupilumab-induced conjunctivitis is based upon severity of presentation. Treatment for very mild conjunctivitis includes topical antihistamines and preservative-free lubrication. Topical calcineurin inhibitors such as tacrolimus or cyclosporine can be considered. Moderate to severe conjunctivitis almost always requires topical corticosteroids. Again, the goal with topical steroid treatment for the indication of dupilumab-induced conjunctivitis is to find the lowest potency and lowest frequency that controls the eye disease. All patients on chronic steroid therapy require ophthalmic monitoring. When atopic eyelid and ocular disease persists dramatically on dupilumab despite dermatitis improvement elsewhere on the body, consideration should be made for patch testing with specific attention to fragrances, preservatives, facial products, and cosmetics. Dupilumab does not appear to suppress patch test reactivity, and identification and elimination of triggers of concomitant atopic contact dermatitis can further help with clinical improvement [20]. Consideration of dupilumab discontinuation should made when atopic conjunctivitis is refractory to topical treatment, if the patient has uncontrolled glaucoma and is not a candidate for topical steroid, or if the reaction is severe such as with cicatricial conjunctivitis. In these instances, strong consideration for alternative systemic agents should be considered. Alternative agents for atopic dermatitis include tralokinumab and upadacitinib. Tralokinumab is a human monoclonal antibody that binds to IL-13. In clinical trials, patients on tralokinumab reported a lower incidence (7.5%) for conjunctivitis compared to dupilumab, but still higher than in the placebo population (3.2%) [21]. This is possibly due to its isolated effect on IL-13 and not both IL-4 and IL-13 as dupilumab. In tralokinumab trials, most cases of conjunctivitis were reported as mild, but were not confirmed as such by ophthalmologic examinations. Upadacitinib, a JAK inhibitor, was also reported to have a lower incidence of conjunctivitis (1.4%) as compared to dupilumab (8.4%) in clinical trials [22].

**Board Review Question Explanation**

Which findings increase the likelihood of dupilumab-induced conjunctivitis?

A. Asthma in addition to dermatitis
B. History of conjunctivitis and more severe baseline dermatitis (correct)
C. Chronic eye rubbing behavior
D. Steroid-dependent atopic dermatitis
E. History of contact lens use

Explanation: **B.** Risk factors for the development of conjunctivitis are prior history of conjunctivitis and more severe baseline systemic dermatitis [5].

**Key Takeaway Points**

- Atopy and atopy-related eye rubbing are associated with vision-threatening complications, such as corneal scarring, cataracts, keratoconus, and retinal detachment.
- Conjunctivitis can be a side effect of dupilumab. Risk factors for occurrence are pre-existing conjunctivitis and/or a severe grade of pre-existing atopic dermatitis.
- Topical corticosteroids can be used safely for the treatment of atopic eye disease and dupilumab-induced conjunctivitis. However, regular ophthalmic monitoring including eye pressure measurement is critical for all patients on chronic recurring steroid therapy to monitor for ocular side effects such as glaucoma and cataract.

## References

1. Iwamoto K, Moriwaki M, Miyake R, Hide M. *Staphylococcus aureus* in atopic dermatitis: strain-specific cell wall proteins and skin immunity. Allergol Int. 2019;68(3):309–15. https://doi.org/10.1016/j.alit.2019.02.006.
2. Borkar DS, Gonzales JA, Tham VM, et al. Association between atopy and herpetic eye disease: results from the pacific ocular inflammation study. JAMA Ophthalmol. 2014;132(3):326–31. https://doi.org/10.1001/jamaophthalmol.2013.6277.
3. Ben-Eli H, Erdinest N, Solomon A. Pathogenesis and complications of chronic eye rubbing in ocular allergy. Curr Opin Allergy Clin Immunol. 2019;19(5):526–34. https://doi.org/10.1097/ACI.0000000000000571.

4. Sahebjada S, Al-Mahrouqi HH, Moshegov S, et al. Eye rubbing in the aetiology of keratoconus: a systematic review and meta-analysis. Graefes Arch Clin Exp Ophthalmol. 2021;259(8):2057–67. https://doi.org/10.1007/s00417-021-05081-8.
5. Akinlade B, Guttman-Yassky E, de Bruin-Weller M, et al. Conjunctivitis in dupilumab clinical trials. Br J Dermatol. 2019;181(3):459–73. https://doi.org/10.1111/bjd.17869.
6. Simpson EL, Bieber T, Guttman-Yassky E, et al. Two phase 3 trials of dupilumab versus placebo in atopic dermatitis. N Engl J Med. 2016;375(24):2335–48. https://doi.org/10.1056/NEJMoa1610020.
7. Wenzel S, Castro M, Corren J, et al. Dupilumab efficacy and safety in adults with uncontrolled persistent asthma despite use of medium-to-high-dose inhaled corticosteroids plus a long-acting beta 2 agonist: a randomised double-blind placebo-controlled pivotal phase 2b dose-ranging trial. Lancet. 2016;388(10039):31–44. https://doi.org/10.1016/S0140-6736(16)30307-5.
8. Rabe KF, Nair P, Brusselle G, et al. Efficacy and safety of dupilumab in glucocorticoid-dependent severe asthma. N Engl J Med. 2018;378(26):2475–85. https://doi.org/10.1056/NEJMoa1804093.
9. Bohner A, Topham C, Strunck J, et al. Dupilumab-associated ocular surface disease: clinical characteristics, treatment, and follow-up. Cornea. 2021;40(5):584–9. https://doi.org/10.1097/ICO.0000000000002461.
10. Gonzalez-Lopez JJ, Lopez-Alcalde J, Morcillo Laiz R, Fernandez Buenaga R, Rebolleda FG. Topical cyclosporine for atopic keratoconjunctivitis. Cochrane Database Syst Rev. 2012;9:CD009078. https://doi.org/10.1002/14651858.CD009078.pub2.
11. Hsu JI, Pflugfelder SC, Kim SJ. Ocular complications of atopic dermatitis. Cutis. 2019;104(3):189–93.
12. Sasoh M, Mizutani H, Matsubara H, et al. Incidence of retinal detachment associated with atopic dermatitis in Japan: review of cases from 1992 to 2011. Clin Ophthalmol. 2015;9:1129–34. https://doi.org/10.2147/OPTH.S85020.
13. Lee Y, Park WK, Kim RY, Kim M, Park YG, Park YH. Characteristics of retinal detachment associated with atopic dermatitis. BMC Ophthalmol. 2021;21(1):359. https://doi.org/10.1186/s12886-021-02135-7.
14. Hashemi H, Heydarian S, Hooshmand E, et al. The prevalence and risk factors for keratoconus: a systematic review and meta-analysis. Cornea. 2020;39(2):263–70. https://doi.org/10.1097/ICO.0000000000002150.
15. Beck KM, Seitzman GD, Yang EJ, Sanchez IM, Liao W. Ocular co-morbidities of atopic dermatitis. Part II: ocular disease secondary to treatments. Am J Clin Dermatol. 2019;20(6):807–15. https://doi.org/10.1007/s40257-019-00465-3.
16. Treister AD, Kraff-Cooper C, Lio PA. Risk factors for dupilumab-associated conjunctivitis in patients with atopic dermatitis. JAMA Dermatol. 2018;154(10):1208–11. https://doi.org/10.1001/jamadermatol.2018.2690.
17. Wollenberg A, Ariens L, Thurau S, van Luijk C, Seegraber M, de Bruin-Weller M. Conjunctivitis occurring in atopic dermatitis patients treated with dupilumab-clinical characteristics and treatment. J Allergy Clin Immunol Pract. 2018;6(5):1778–1780 e1. https://doi.org/10.1016/j.jaip.2018.01.034.
18. Reddy AK, Hauswirth SG, Gregory DG, Liao SD, Palestine AG. Dupilumab-associated cicatrizing ocular disease. Am J Ophthalmol Case Rep. 2022;26:101528. https://doi.org/10.1016/j.ajoc.2022.101528.
19. Nguyen MT, Tsukikawa M, Lomazow W, Lee M. Irreversible bilateral cicatricial keratoconjunctivitis after dupilumab therapy. Case Rep Ophthalmol. 2022;13(2):638–42. https://doi.org/10.1159/000525738.
20. Raffi J, Suresh R, Botto N, Murase JE. The impact of dupilumab on patch testing and the prevalence of comorbid allergic contact dermatitis in recalcitrant atopic dermatitis: a retrospective chart review. J Am Acad Dermatol. 2020;82(1):132–8. https://doi.org/10.1016/j.jaad.2019.09.028.

21. Wollenberg A, Beck LA, de Bruin WM, et al. Conjunctivitis in adult patients with moderate-to-severe atopic dermatitis: results from five tralokinumab clinical trials. Br J Dermatol. 2022;186(3):453–65. https://doi.org/10.1111/bjd.20810.
22. Blauvelt A, Teixeira HD, Simpson EL, et al. Efficacy and safety of upadacitinib vs dupilumab in adults with moderate-to-severe atopic dermatitis: a randomized clinical trial. JAMA Dermatol. 2021;157(9):1047–55. https://doi.org/10.1001/jamadermatol.2021.3023.

# Chapter 12
# Management of Facial Erythema on Dupilumab Treatment

**Kripa Ahuja and Peter Lio**

**Case Title** "A 45-year-old female presents with a fine, scaling, edematous rash."

**Case**
It's Monday morning, and your first patient of the day is a middle-aged woman who presents with a 2-week history of a "pink, scaly rash." The eruption is mildly edematous and erythematous, with pink and red plaques. The rash is concentrated on the face and neck, particularly the anterolateral neck and periocular face. Upon asking the patient about her previous medical history, you learn she has a long history of moderate atopic dermatitis, for which she was started on dupilumab 6 months prior to the visit. The patient also has a past medical history of type 2 diabetes mellitus and hypertension and is currently managed with several medications. You have a medical student doing a dermatology rotation with you. He asks you what you suspect the cause of the patient's facial erythema is. How do you respond to this medical student?

**Board Review Question**
Which of the following medications are associated with facial erythema?

A. Dupilumab
B. Topical calcineurin inhibitors
C. Metformin
D. ACE inhibitors
E. A and B
F. C and D
G. All of the above

K. Ahuja
Eastern Virginia Medical School, Norfolk, VA, USA
e-mail: AhujaK@evms.edu

P. Lio (✉)
Northwestern University Feinberg School of Medicine, Chicago, IL, USA



N. Brownstone et al. (eds.), *Clinical Cases in Atopic Dermatitis*, Clinical Cases in Dermatology, https://doi.org/10.1007/978-3-031-52147-8_12

## Overview of Atopic Dermatitis

Atopic dermatitis (AD) is a chronic relapsing and remitting disorder prevalent across all ages, severely reducing the quality of life. The cornerstone of AD treatment has long been topical corticosteroids (TCS). However, prolonged use of these drugs, particularly on the face and neck, is not recommended. In the past several years, non-steroidal therapies have been developed that show great promise in treating AD. One of these agents, dupilumab, was approved by the US Food and Drug Administration (FDA) in 2017. Dupilumab has made great strides in reducing flares, decreasing symptoms, and overall improving the quality of life in patients with AD, demonstrated by multiple studies and clinical trials.

The proinflammatory cytokines interleukin-4 (IL-4) and interleukin-13 (IL-13) are at the center of the pathophysiology of AD. Dupilumab is a monoclonal antibody of the immunoglobulin G4 subclass that inhibits IL-4 and IL-13 signaling by binding to the IL-4 receptor alpha subunit, which both IL-4 and IL-13 share in their respective receptor signaling. By blocking IL-4 and IL-13 signaling, dupilumab inhibits the cytokine-induced response of release of proinflammatory cytokines, vasodilation, and immunoglobulin E (IgE) production.

The most common reported adverse events of dupilumab are injection site reactions, herpes simplex infections, headaches, and nasopharyngitis. Additionally, dupilumab has an associated ocular surface disease, particularly conjunctivitis, but also blepharitis, keratitis, eye pruritus, and dry eye.

A more recently described side effect is the development of facial erythema after dupilumab treatment. This side effect was initially reported in 2018 in a Caucasian woman. After initial improvement on the drug, the patient developed a worsening rash on her face and neck. Skin biopsy showed spongiotic dermatitis. Laboratory workup was non-contributory, and various topical preparations, such as calcipotriene, oxiconazole, topical ivermectin, and topical clobetasol, failed to provide relief. Since then, many other cases of drug-associated face and neck dermatitis (DAFND) have been reported, though it is difficult to estimate the incidence.

## Presentation of DAFND

The presentation of DAFND is not uniform and may represent multiple distinct entities. In some cases, dermatitis presents only a week after injection, while it may take 5 or 6 months in other cases. Many patients have ocular symptoms, predominantly conjunctivitis, along with dermatitis, but eye symptoms are not invariable. In some instances, the dermatitis may initially appear to be an exacerbation of the patient's underlying AD, while others report distinctive morphology, distribution, and/or symptomatology from their previous skin condition.

## Proposed Pathophysiology of DAFND

The underlying mechanism for DAFND remains to be elucidated. However, there are several theories that may help organize thinking about the condition.

## Inhibition of Th2 Cells

Dupilumab inhibits IL-4 and IL-13, ultimately blocking the Th2 cellular pathway. There have been some case studies describing DAFND presenting in a rosacea-like fashion, with other case studies describing patients developing psoriasis after dupilumab initiation. Because both rosacea and psoriasis involve Th1 and Th17 pathways, there is speculation that suppressing Th2 cells leads to overactivation of the Th1 and Th17 pathways. Additionally, an increased colonization of the follicular *Demodex* mite has also been proposed as a possible DAFND pathophysiology. In mice, impairing Th2 cells has led to proliferation of *Demodex* mites.

Hypersensitivity to the fungus *Malassezia* is another possible pathophysiology for DAFND because elevated serum levels of *Malassezia*-specific IgE levels have been found in patients presenting with DAFND, with subsequent clearance of the DAFND with the antifungal drug itraconazole. The weakened skin barrier in patients with AD permits easier colonization of *Malassezia*. Furthermore, mouse models have shown that *Malassezia* selectively induces Th17-based inflammation, a possible explanation for some patients' stronger responses against *Malassezia* that could have resulted from Th2 suppression due to dupilumab.

Speculatively, the dysfunctional balance of helper T cells might explain the development of certain allergens after dupilumab use. The development of anti-drug antibodies as in the case of other biological agents is another possible pathophysiology, though once again hypothetical.

## Differential Diagnosis of New Facial Erythema and Eruption on Dupilumab

The nosology of erythematous rashes on the face and neck in the setting of dupilumab may be due to multiple possible etiologies. Because of this, clinicians must employ different diagnostic tools to identify the offending rash. When faced with a patient who presents with facial erythema after starting dupilumab, the provider should first take a complete history and review medications to rule out any other drugs that could be the culprit (e.g., metformin, ACE inhibitors, and various other drugs have been associated with facial erythema). The provider should ascertain if there have been any changes in the patient's life that could have provoked the rash (diet, routine, soap, etc.). Once a thorough history and timeline have been established, the provider is ready to move forward with possible differential diagnoses.

The differential diagnosis for DAFND is fairly extensive and includes allergic contact dermatitis (ACD), rosacea/steroid-induced rosacea (SIR), periorificial dermatitis (POD), demodicosis, topical steroid withdrawal syndrome (TSWS), *Malassezia* head and neck dermatitis, photodermatitis, seborrheic dermatitis, psoriasis, and more. (Please see Table 12.1.)

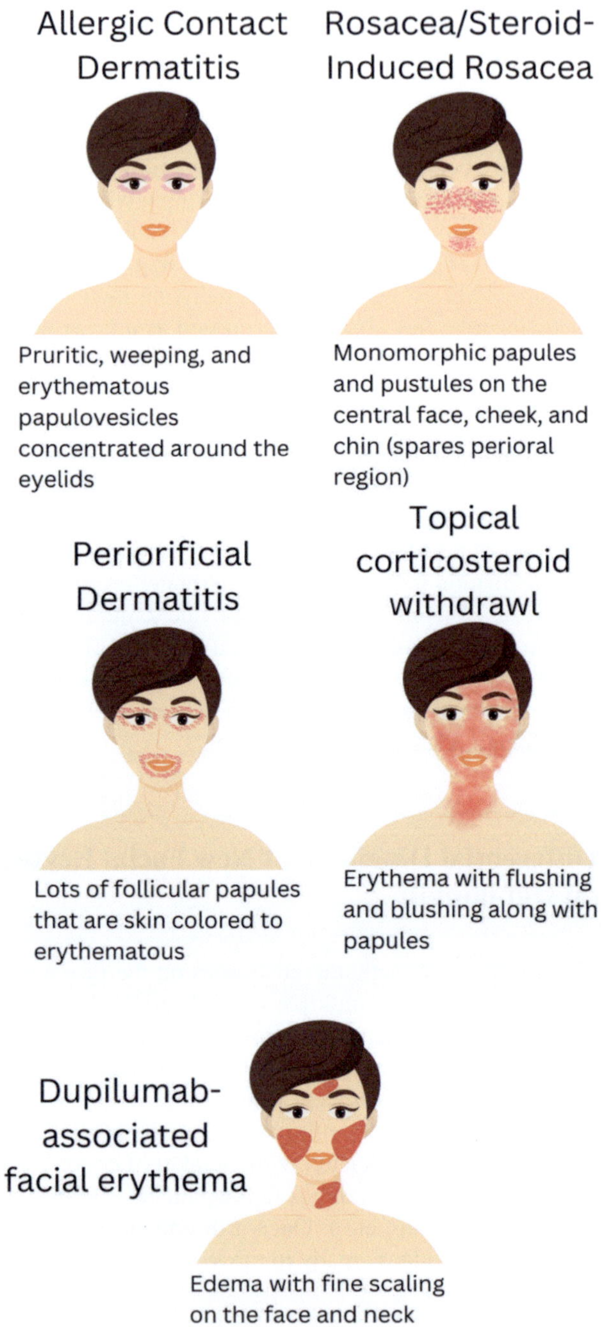


**Fig. 12.1** Illustration of selected facial and neck dermatoses

**Table 12.1** Selected cases of facial and neck dermatitis post dupilumab use

| Patient's age and sex | Skin biopsy | Dupilumab use (previous, continued) | Adverse effect (rash description, location, ocular symptoms) | Relevant medical history | Patch testing | References |
|---|---|---|---|---|---|---|
| 26, female | Spongiotic dermatitis | 6 months, stopped | Face, anterolateral neck, fine scaling, edematous, pink red, plaques | Positive ANA: 1:160 (homogeneous, speckled) | Not performed | Dalia Y, Johnson SM. Case report: First reported case of facial rash after dupilumab therapy. Pract Dermatol. 2018;25–26 |
| 26, female | Not performed | 7 months, stopped | Pruritic rash on upper and lower eyelids (prior to dupilumab treatment) worsened to involve arms | N/A | +/– Carba mix and lanolin<br>1+ triethanolamine<br>3+ bacitracin and neomycin | Hoot JW, Douglas JD, Falo LD Jr. patch testing in a patient on dupilumab. Dermatitis. 2018;29(3):164. Doi: 10.1097/DER.0000000000000357. PMID: 29570490 |
| 52, female | Not performed | Allergen testing and subsequent avoidance improved rash, patient still on dupilumab | Previous dermatitis persisted on the face, neck, and forearms | N/A | –/2+ neomycin sulfate 20%<br>–/2+ bacitracin 20%<br>Trace/2+ ethyl acrylate 0.1%<br>1+/2+ glutaraldehyde 1%<br>–/2+ ammonium persulfate 2.5% | Suresh R, Murase JE. The role of expanded series patch testing in identifying causality of residual facial dermatitis following initiation of dupilumab therapy. JAAD Case Rep. 2018;4(9):899–904 |

(continued)

**Table 12.1** (continued)

| Patient's age and sex | Skin biopsy | Dupilumab use (previous, continued) | Adverse effect (rash description, location, ocular symptoms) | Relevant medical history | Patch testing | References |
|---|---|---|---|---|---|---|
| 54, female | Not done | Allergen testing and subsequent avoidance was successful, patient still on dupilumab | Dupilumab improved overall rash; facial rash persisted | Not done | Allergies to budesonide, alclometasone, and limonene | Suresh R, Murase JE. The role of expanded series patch testing in identifying causality of residual facial dermatitis following initiation of dupilumab therapy. JAAD Case Rep. 2018;4(9):899–904 |
| 54, female | Not done | No rash following dupilumab; dupilumab cleared facial rash | Mild generalized pruritus on the face | Not done | Sweet baby shampoo | Suresh R, Murase JE. The role of expanded series patch testing in identifying causality of residual facial dermatitis following initiation of dupilumab therapy. JAAD Case Rep. 2018;4(9):899–904 |

| | | | | | | |
|---|---|---|---|---|---|---|
| 66, female | Not done | Seven days after her first and only dupilumab injection, rash resolved 12.5 weeks after dupilumab injection | Severe periocular dermatitis, unlike previous AD symptoms, with exacerbation of her perioral AD<br>Severe periocular erythema with skin thickening, peeling, and secondary ectropion<br>Upon examination 3 weeks later, the patient's periocular dermatitis now extended to the lateral temples and was nearly confluent over the bridge of her nose (Fig. 12.1). Anterior segment examination showed diffuse 1+ chemosis and 2+ conjunctival injection OU | Past ophthalmic history was pertinent for bilateral upper and lower lid blepharoplasty 14 years prior to presentation. At presentation, a slit lamp examination was positive only for trace inferior injection and rare superficial punctate keratitis bilaterally | Allergy to benzalkonium chloride | Yamane MLM, Belsito DV, Glass LRD. Two differing presentations of periocular dermatitis as a side effect of dupilumab for atopic dermatitis. Orbit. 2019;38(5):390–394 |

(continued)

**Table 12.1** (continued)

| Patient's age and sex | Skin biopsy | Dupilumab use (previous, continued) | Adverse effect (rash description, location, ocular symptoms) | Relevant medical history | Patch testing | References |
|---|---|---|---|---|---|---|
| 28, female | Not done | After 11 dupilumab injections (5.5 months), periocular dermatitis fully resolved within 13 weeks | Periocular dermatitis, eye redness, excess tearing, and a raised rash around her eyes. For 2 days prior to presentation, the patient experienced yellowish discharge OU and awoke with her eyes crusted and glued shut | External examination was significant for bilateral periocular erythema and edema, most prominent at the medial aspect of her eyelids, with bilateral upper and lower skin crease thickening. She had a fine, erythematous rash at her lateral canthi and nose, consistent with her other eczema sites. Slit lamp examination showed mild conjunctival injection and intense pre-tarsal papillary reaction of the upper and lower lids OU. She was diagnosed with bilateral periocular dermatitis and conjunctivitis in the setting of dupilumab use | Pimecrolimus, chromium, nickel, ragweed, trees, and ibuprofen | Yamane MLM, Belsito DV, Glass LRD. Two differing presentations of periocular dermatitis as a side effect of dupilumab for atopic dermatitis. Orbit. 2019;38(5):390–394 |

| | | | | | | |
|---|---|---|---|---|---|---|
| 61, male | Not done | Two months after starting, patient continued on it;<br>4 months later, had progressive ocular symptoms; and stopped dupilumab. Ocular symptoms normalized but AD returned | Noted eyelid redness, crusting, tearing, and intermittent blurred vision | Previous medical history significant for systemic immunosuppressive therapy for AD. On presentation, best corrected visual acuity was 20/30 in each eye. Intraocular pressure was normal and there was no afferent pupillary defect. External examination revealed severe cicatricial ectropion with punctal stenosis of both lower eyelids, hyperemic eyelid margins, and significant conjunctival injection that extended beyond the interpalpebral zone of both eyes. Dilation and irrigation of both lower punctae showed moderate punctal stenosis | Not done | Barnes AC, Blandford AD, Perry JD. Cicatricial ectropion in a patient treated with dupilumab. Am J Ophthalmol Case Rep. 2017;7:120–2. |

## Allergic Contact Dermatitis

Many patients with AD have a pre-existing impaired epidermal barrier making them more susceptible to antigen entry into the skin with subsequent sensitization. Allergic contact dermatitis (ACD) generally presents as an erythematous, eczematous, or vesicular dermatitis typically localized to the skin area that was exposed to the allergen. This dermatitis can have crusted or weeping lesions and can become more lichenified in chronic cases. A skin biopsy will often reveal spongiosis, but may not be entirely specific.

Allergen patch testing is generally considered the gold standard in the diagnosis of ACD. While there is some debate about whether or not dupilumab can affect patch test results, pragmatically, if an allergen is driving the facial dermatitis, it is likely to be positive on patch testing despite any immunomodulatory effect of the dupilumab. If an allergen is identified, careful avoidance of the allergen and its cross reactants is generally curative, though it may take weeks or even months to fully resolve. More acutely, compresses with black tea have been demonstrated to quickly improve facial dermatitis (both AD and allergic contact dermatitis were included in the study), and topical corticosteroids or non-steroidal agents may be useful to cool inflammation and expedite healing.

## Topical Steroid Withdrawal Syndrome

Topical steroid withdrawal syndrome (TSWS) is an incompletely understood phenomenon that presents with erythema, burning, and/or itching generally after chronic use of higher-potency topical and/or systemic corticosteroids. TSWS often presents on the face and neck making it an important diagnostic consideration.

As topical steroids are a cornerstone of AD treatment, most patients who present with DAFND have likely been exposed to topical and/or oral steroids for months or years. At this time, lacking clear diagnostic criteria means that clinicians may have to rely on a *diagnosis ex juvantibus* approach: specifically, stopping the dupilumab to see if that improves that eruption would most convincingly differentiate between these two entities.

## Rosacea/Steroid-Induced Rosacea and Demodicosis

Steroid-induced rosacea (SIR) is associated with use of topical steroids on the face. Vasomotor instability is part of the proposed pathophysiology. SIR is clinically indistinguishable from classical rosacea, which presents on the forehead, nose, and cheeks with erythematous monomorphic papules or pustules on an erythematous and sometimes edematous background. There is a somewhat confusing overlap with demodicosis, with many feeling that these are closely related conditions.

Characteristic morphology, personal or family history, and sometimes simply empirically to see if it responds to appropriate therapy (*diagnosis ex juvantibus*) may help make the diagnosis. Topical therapy with metronidazole, ivermectin, or azelaic acid (and combinations thereof) may be used as first line. In more severe or refractory cases, oral therapy with tetracycline antibiotics generally leads to significant improvement. For some, lifestyle and environmental management will need to be continued (along with medications at times) as rosacea can be chronic.

## Periorificial Dermatitis

Periorificial dermatitis is in many ways similar to rosacea. Like rosacea, it may also be steroid-induced. Even inhaled corticosteroids for asthma (particularly in younger children who use a face mask) can be a culprit. Differentiating it from rosacea is the focus around the mouth, nose, and eyes, but management is essentially the same as for rosacea. For many, however, it can be refractory to topical therapy, and oral antibiotics of the tetracycline class tend to be most useful. Topical calcineurin inhibitors may also improve clearance in difficult cases.

## Malassezia

As mentioned in the proposed pathophysiology for DAFND, another possible is an immune response to *Malassezia. Malassezia* is a yeast that is a part of normal skin flora and is found in skin areas that are rich in sebaceous glands, such as the head and neck. *Malassezia* also more commonly occurs in hot and humid environments, often seen in athletes who spend long periods of time in the sun. It typically presents with erythematous and scaling patches, sometimes itchy. Differentiation of *Malassezia* from rosacea involves significant pruritus. Confirmation of *Malassezia* can be made via KOH preparation, although in this context the sensitivity of this test is unclear.

## Management for DAFND

Some evidence has demonstrated that DAFND may respond to short courses of low- to mid-potency topical corticosteroids (TCS), topical calcineurin inhibitors (TCIs), and/or topical and/or systemic azole antifungals without stopping dupilumab. For milder symptoms, topical emollients may be sufficient. For more moderate cases, systemic therapies including prednisone, itraconazole, doxycycline, or antihistamines can be used. If the patient does not respond to the stepwise approach or has severe symptoms, systemic methotrexate, cyclosporine, or discontinuation of dupilumab may also be considered. Clinicians should use their best clinical determination and consult with other physicians as necessary for the best course of action.

## Patient Education

Because of the heterogeneity in possible diagnoses, workup and empiric therapy should be initiated promptly. When suspected to be drug related and not responding to therapies, the dupilumab should be held if possible or replaced with another agent.

**Board Review Question Explanation**
Which of the following medications are associated with facial erythema?

A. Dupilumab.
B. Topical calcineurin inhibitors.
C. Metformin.
D. ACE inhibitors.
E. A and B.
F. C and D.
G. All of the above (correct).

Explanation: Dupilumab, topical calcineurin inhibitors, metformin, and ACE inhibitors all have been associated with facial erythema, facial angioedema, and facial flushing.

**Key Takeaway Points**

- Dupilumab is a biologic agent used to treat AD by inhibiting IL-4 and IL-13.
- A reported adverse effect of dupilumab is facial erythema.
- The facial erythema presentation is somewhat variable: the rash can present after a week or many months, can include conjunctivitis and ocular symptoms, and may be difficult to distinguish from other causes of facial dermatitis.
- Allergic contact dermatitis is an important possible cause that must be carefully evaluated.
- Patch testing may prove beneficial in such cases, but other entities must be considered including drug-induced.

## Further Reading

1. Jaros J, Hendricks AJ, Shi VY, Lio PA. A practical approach to recalcitrant face and neck dermatitis in atopic dermatitis. Dermatitis. 2020;31(3):169–77. https://doi.org/10.1097/DER.0000000000000590.
2. Din ATU, Malik I, Arshad D, Din ATU. Dupilumab for atopic dermatitis: the silver bullet we have been searching for? Cureus. 2020;12(4):e7565. https://doi.org/10.7759/cureus.7565.

3. D'Ippolito D, Pisano M. Dupilumab (Dupixent): an interleukin-4 receptor antagonist for atopic dermatitis. P T. 2018;43(9):532–5. PMID: 30186024; PMCID: PMC6110636.
4. DUPIXENT (Dupilumab). injection-Accessdata.fda.gov. https://www.accessdata.fda.gov/drugsatfda_docs/label/2017/761053lbl.pdf. Accessed 25 Aug 2022.
5. Dalia Y, Johnson SM. Case report: first reported case of facial rash after dupilumab therapy. Pract Dermatol. 2018;15:25–6.
6. Hoot JW, Douglas JD, Falo LD Jr. Patch testing in a patient on dupilumab. Dermatitis. 2018;29(3):164. https://doi.org/10.1097/DER.0000000000000357.
7. Suresh R, Murase JE. The role of expanded series patch testing in identifying causality of residual facial dermatitis following initiation of dupilumab therapy. JAAD Case Rep. 2018;4(9):899–904.
8. Yamane MLM, Belsito DV, Glass LRD. Two differing presentations of periocular dermatitis as a side effect of dupilumab for atopic dermatitis. Orbit. 2019;38(5):390–4.
9. Barnes AC, Blandford AD, Perry JD. Cicatricial ectropion in a patient treated with dupilumab. Am J Ophthalmol Case Rep. 2017;7:120–2.
10. Zhu GA, Chen JK, Chiou A, et al. New regional dermatoses during dupilumab therapy for atopic dermatitis. J Invest Dermatol. 2019;139(5):535.
11. Muzumdar S, Skudalski L, Sharp K, Waldman RA. Dupilumab facial redness/dupilumab facial dermatitis: a guide for clinicians. Am J Clin Dermatol. 2022;23(1):61–7. https://doi.org/10.1007/s40257-021-00646-z. Epub 2021 Dec 2.
12. Maarouf M, Saberian C, Lio PA, Shi VY. Head-and-neck dermatitis: diagnostic difficulties and management pearls. Pediatr Dermatol. 2018;35(6):748–53. https://doi.org/10.1111/pde.13642. Epub 2018 Aug 28.
13. Patruno C, Amerio P, Chiricozzi A, Costanzo A, Cristaudo A, Cusano F, Foti C, Girolomoni G, Guarneri F, Naldi L, Offidani A, Pigatto P, Prignano F, Stingeni L, Calzavara-Pinton P. Optimizing a clinical guidance for diagnosis of atopic dermatitis in adults: joint recommendations of the Italian Society of Dermatology and Venereology (SIDeMaST), Italian Association of Hospital Dermatologists (ADOI), and Italian Society of Allergological, Occupational and Environmental Dermatology (SIDAPA). G Ital Dermatol Venereol. 2020;155(1):1–7. https://doi.org/10.23736/S0392-0488.19.06522-2. Epub 2019 Dec 16.
14. Murphy PB, Atwater AR, Mueller M. Allergic contact dermatitis. In: StatPearls. Treasure Island (FL): StatPearls Publishing; 2022. https://www.ncbi.nlm.nih.gov/books/NBK532866/.
15. Hwang J, Lio PA. Topical corticosteroid withdrawal ("steroid addiction"): an update of a systematic review. J Dermatol Treat. 2021;33:1293. https://doi.org/10.1080/09546634.2021.1882659.
16. Sheary B. Topical steroid withdrawal: a case series of 10 children. Acta Derm Venereol. 2019;99(6):551–6. https://doi.org/10.2340/00015555-3144.
17. Lio P, Chandan N. Topical steroid withdrawal in atopic dermatitis. Pract Dermatol. https://practicaldermatology.com/articles/2019-aug/topical-steroid-withdrawal-in-atopic-dermatitis. Accessed 28 July 2022.
18. Tolaymat L, Hall MR. Perioral dermatitis. In: StatPearls. Treasure Island (FL): StatPearls Publishing; 2022. https://www.ncbi.nlm.nih.gov/books/NBK525968/.
19. Hsu FO. Case study: Lip swelling and herbal medicine. Amethyst Holistic Skin Solutions. https://amethystacu.com/case-study-lip-swelling-and-herbal-medicine/. Accessed 28 July 2022.
20. Jo CE, Finstad A, Georgakopoulos JR, Piguet V, Yeung J, Drucker AM. Facial and neck erythema associated with dupilumab treatment: a systematic review. J Am Acad Dermatol. 2021;84(5):1339–47. https://doi.org/10.1016/j.jaad.2021.01.012. Epub 2021 Jan 8.
21. de Beer FSA, Bakker DS, Haeck I, Ariens L, van der Schaft J, van Dijk MR, de Bruin-Weller MS. Dupilumab facial redness: positive effect of itraconazole. JAAD Case Rep. 2019;5(10):888–91. https://doi.org/10.1016/j.jdcr.2019.07.020.
22. Vest BE, Krauland K. *Malassezia furfur*. In: StatPearls. Treasure Island (FL): StatPearls Publishing; 2022. https://www.ncbi.nlm.nih.gov/books/NBK553091/.

23. Papp KA, Hong C, Lansang MP, et al. Practical management of patients with atopic dermatitis on dupilumab. Dermatol Ther (Heidelb). 2021;11:1805–28. https://doi.org/10.1007/s13555-021-00586-w.
24. Gooderham M, McDonald J, Papp K. Diagnosis and management of conjunctivitis for the dermatologist. J Cutan Med Surg. 2018;22(2):200–6. https://doi.org/10.1177/1203475417743233. Epub 2017 Dec 1.
25. Witte M, Krause L, Zillikens D, Shimanovich I. Black tea dressings—a rapidly effective treatment for facial dermatitis. J Dermatol Treat. 2019;30:785. https://doi.org/10.1080/09546634.2019.1573306.

# Chapter 13
# Treatment of Erythrodermic Atopic Dermatitis with Cyclosporine

**Katie Roster, Madison Hackley, Nicholas Brownstone, and John Koo**

**Case Title** A 40-year-old man with widespread erythema of the skin.

**Case**
A 40-year-old man comes to your office with widespread skin erythema covering 80% of his body. The skin has become scaly and thickened, and he says he has been unable to sleep for the last few days due to the pain and pruritus. You diagnose him with erythrodermic atopic dermatitis and consider systemic therapies that will act quickly and effectively to treat this patient's condition.

**Board Review Question**
A 43-year-old woman comes to the physician for severe atopic dermatitis. Her pulse is 80/min, and her blood pressure is 130/70 mmHg. She has been using topical triamcinolone 0.1% for her rash. The physician recommends a systemic treatment that works rapidly, is well-tolerated in the short term, and is likely to quickly be approved by insurance. The recommended agent dampens the T-cell response by decreasing cytokine transcription. Which of the following should be performed before initiating this medication?

K. Roster
New York Medical College, Valhalla, NY, USA

M. Hackley
Temple University Lewis Katz School of Medicine, Philadelphia, PA, USA
e-mail: madison.hackley@temple.edu

N. Brownstone
Department of Dermatology, Temple University Hospital, Philadelphia, PA, USA

J. Koo (✉)
Department of Dermatology, University of California, San Francisco,
San Francisco, PA, USA



N. Brownstone et al. (eds.), *Clinical Cases in Atopic Dermatitis*, Clinical Cases in Dermatology, https://doi.org/10.1007/978-3-031-52147-8_13

A. Pulmonary function test
B. Eye examination
C. Creatinine measurement
D. Discontinuation of topical treatment

## Main Text

Erythrodermic atopic dermatitis and severe atopic dermatitis (AD) can be managed with high-potency topical corticosteroids or oral corticosteroids. Patients who have relapsed or have failed to respond to these first-line agents can be treated with immunosuppressants or immunomodulators such as methotrexate, azathioprine, dupilumab, or cyclosporine.

Cyclosporine A (CsA) is an effective and fast-acting treatment for inflammatory skin disorders including erythrodermic AD, severe AD, and psoriasis. Studies have shown symptoms begin to improve in as little as 1 week, and up to 90% of patients achieve clearance or significant improvement [1–4]. Cyclosporine has also been shown to have a decreased incidence of rebound symptoms when compared to corticosteroids [1].

Cyclosporine works by binding with cyclophilin to inhibit calcineurin and the nuclear factor of activated T-cells (NFAT). The inhibition of NFAT decreases the production of various cytokines, such as IL-2, and decreases the expression of the IL-2 receptors. Consequently, the number of differentiated and activated T cells declines [4]. This rapid suppression of the cell-mediated immune response makes cyclosporine a powerful drug for treating T-cell-driven diseases such as atopic dermatitis [4–6].

Several clinical trials have evaluated the effectiveness of cyclosporine for atopic dermatitis. A 2013 systematic review of several clinical trials evaluated the efficacy of cyclosporine. Five clinical trials found that cyclosporine is superior to placebo [2]. Additional clinical trials concluded that cyclosporine is more effective than prednisone, IVIG, and UVAB for treating atopic dermatitis [1–3, 5, 7, 8].

Despite these benefits, cyclosporine is typically reserved for severe, treatment-resistant atopic dermatitis and is not suitable for long-term use [5]. Long-term use of cyclosporine has been associated with hypertension, gingival hyperplasia, hirsutism, nephrotoxicity, hyperlipidemia, and hyperglycemia [9–12]. The most common side effects associated with cyclosporine are neurologic and can occur in patients even when cyclosporine is used for only a short period of time. These neurological symptoms include tremors, headaches, paresthesia, and hyperesthesia. Note, however, that tremor is a relatively rare side effect in dermatologic patients [9].

Like other immunosuppressive drugs, cyclosporine can cause myalgias and malaise and increases one's susceptibility to infections [9]. Patients should be made aware that cyclosporine is associated with an increased risk of non-melanoma skin cancer (NMSC) [13]. There is also an association with internal cancers. However, these associations are more of a concern with the high doses of cyclosporine typically given to organ transplant patients [9, 10, 12, 13].

Before starting patients on cyclosporine, it is important to conduct a physical exam, obtain a thorough history, and run several laboratory tests. Cyclosporine is contraindicated in patients with uncontrolled hypertension or abnormal renal functions [9, 10]. Current infection or malignancy is also a contraindication to cyclosporine. Before starting cyclosporine, two blood pressure measurements should be taken at least 1 day apart [9, 13, 14]. A complete blood count, complete metabolic panel (including BUN/Cr), and fasting lipid profile are also needed. Uric acid levels should be checked at baseline for patients at risk for gout. Baseline magnesium and potassium should also be checked, given the potential of hypomagnesemia and hyperkalemia (although serum magnesium may not be relevant if cyclosporine is used for a limited duration). Special attention should be given to the creatine and uremic level, as nephrotoxicity is a particular concern with cyclosporine use. For extra precaution, two baseline creatine levels should be taken at least 1 day apart [9].

The recommended starting dose of cyclosporine is 2.5–5 mg/kg daily [9, 12, 15]. When prescribing cyclosporine to obese patients, the starting dose should be based on their ideal body weight instead of their current weight. Cyclosporine is most effective when combined with a topical corticosteroid, so additional topical therapy can be considered. Emollients and oral anti-histamine can be given as well if needed [2, 7]. Due to its association with NMSC, concomitant use of cyclosporine with phototherapy is not advised [9].

After starting therapy, patients must be monitored every 2 weeks for the first 1–2 months. Blood pressure measurement and complete blood count with a BUN/Cr level, CBC, lipids, and uric acid levels should be taken every 2 weeks. Electrolyte levels should be measured to monitor for hypomagnesemia and hyperkalemia. After 12 weeks, patients can transition to monthly lab monitoring (Table 13.1) [2, 9, 13, 14].

**Table 13.1** Lab monitoring of cyclosporine

| Initial tests |
|---|
| Two blood pressure tests at least 1 day apart |
| Two creatinine levels at least 1 day apart |
| Comprehensive metabolic panel (CMP) |
| Complete blood count (CBC) |
| Liver function tests |
| Lipids |
| Magnesium, potassium |
| Uric acid |

| First 1–2 months, every 2 weeks, then monthly |
|---|
| Blood pressure |
| Comprehensive metabolic panel (CMP) |
| Complete blood count (CBC) |
| Lipids |
| Magnesium, potassium |
| Uric acid |

As previously noted, nephrotoxicity is a major complication of cyclosporine use [12]. The dose of cyclosporine must be decreased or discontinued if the patient's creatinine level increases by 30% or more upon two different measurements taken 2 weeks apart. An increase in creatinine of 50% or more also warrants immediate discontinuation until serum creatinine returns to baseline [2, 9, 15].

Patients can be encouraged to monitor their BP at home. If hypertension develops during therapy, the dose can be decreased, or hypertension can be managed with a calcium channel blocker such as nifedipine or isradipine. The development of hyperlipidemia can be treated with lifestyle changes or, if needed, a statin [2, 9].

According to US FDA guidelines, cyclosporine treatment should not exceed 1 year, as long-term use is associated with multiple adverse events, such as nephrotoxicity, neurotoxicity, and dyslipidemia. However, continuous courses of cyclosporine may be used for up to 2 years, according to worldwide consensus guidelines [16, 17]. If a patient's symptoms are well-controlled after 4–12 months of cyclosporine therapy, and symptoms are well-controlled, patients can be transitioned to another immunosuppressive agent such as methotrexate, mycophenolate, azathioprine, or dupilumab [9]. Dupilumab, approved in 2017 for atopic dermatitis, is an effective long-term treatment option for patients due to its high specificity for IL-3 and IL-4 and its limited side effect profile. Dupilumab takes up to 16 weeks to reach full clinical efficacy [8], during which time cyclosporine must be slowly tapered down, as sudden discontinuation can cause a rebound flare of symptoms [7]. Different dosing protocols for the transition from cyclosporine A to dupilumab have been proposed. A safe and general consensus is to reduce the dose by 0.5–1.0 mg/kg/day every 2 weeks until the achievement of clinical benefits (Fig. 13.1) [12]. Ludwig et al. recommend starting dupilumab and continuing the current cyclosporine dose for 3 weeks. After week 3, the dose of cyclosporine can be halved three times over the next 9 weeks [16]. For example, in a patient taking 200 mg daily of cyclosporine, the dose would be lowered to 100 mg, then 50 mg, and then 25 mg at weeks 3, 6, and 9 and then discontinued at week 12 (Table 13.2). The transition to other

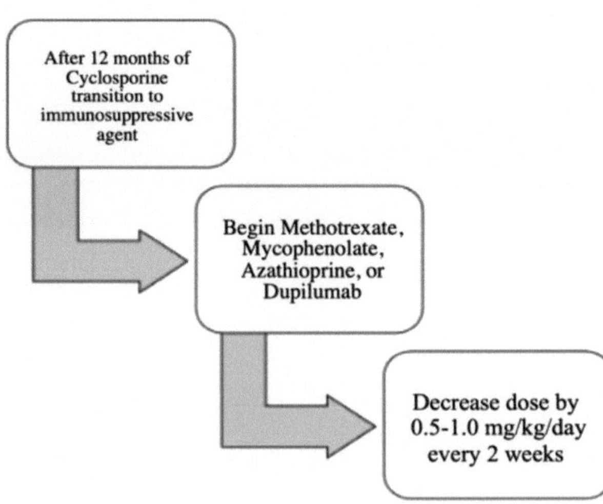


**Fig. 13.1** Proposed method from Megna et al. for transitioning from cyclosporine to other systemic therapy

**Table 13.2** Example of another proposed method by Ludwig et al. of transitioning from cyclosporine to dupilumab

| Week number after starting dupilumab | Cyclosporine dose |
|---|---|
| Week 0 | 200 mg daily |
| Week 3 | 100 mg daily |
| Week 6 | 50 mg daily |
| Week 9 | 25 mg daily |
| Week 12 | 0 mg daily |

immunosuppressives is similar. For example, transitioning to a TNF antagonist or ustekinumab is done with a short overlap period of 2–8 weeks to prevent recurrence in psoriasis patients [18]. During the transition to any immunosuppressive agent, the recommended lab monitoring outlined above should continue.

**Board Review Question Explanation**

A 43-year-old woman comes to the physician for severe atopic dermatitis. Her pulse is 80/min, and her blood pressure is 130/70 mmHg. She has been using topical triamcinolone 0.1% for her rash. The physician recommends a systemic treatment that works rapidly, is well-tolerated in the short term, and is likely to quickly be approved by insurance. The recommended agent dampens the T-cell response by decreasing cytokine transcription. Which of the following should be performed before initiating this medication?

A. Pulmonary function test
B. Eye examination
C. Creatinine measurement (correct)
D. Discontinuation of topical treatment

**Explanation**

The correct answer is C. Creatinine measurement. Initial tests include two blood pressure measurements at least 1 day apart, CMP, CBC, liver function tests, lipids, uric acid levels, and a magnesium/potassium level (Table 13.1). Prescribers should pay special attention to the creatinine level because cyclosporine can cause irreversible kidney damage. Providers must take two baseline creatinine levels at least 1 day apart.

**Key Takeaway Points**

- Cyclosporine inhibits calcineurin to suppress cytokine transcription and suppress T-cells.
- Multiple studies have demonstrated that cyclosporine is highly effective in treating erythrodermic atopic dermatitis and severe atopic dermatitis.
- Despite its benefits when used long term, cyclosporine has a lengthy side effect profile; the most significant concern is renal impairment. Therefore, short-term use of cyclosporine followed by a transition to another agent with a better long-term safety profile is recommended.
- The drug requires frequent lab monitoring every 2 weeks for the first 1–2 months.

## References

1. Nankervis H, Thomas KS, Delamere FM, et al. Scoping systematic review of treatments for eczema (Programme Grants for Applied Research, No. 4.7.). Southampton: NIHR Journals Library; 2016. https://www.ncbi.nlm.nih.gov/books/NBK363127/. https://doi.org/10.3310/pgfar04070.
2. Roekevisch E, Spuls PI, Kuester D, Limpens J, Schmitt J. Efficacy and safety of systemic treatments for moderate-to-severe atopic dermatitis: a systematic review. J Allergy Clin Immunol. 2014;133(2):429–38. https://doi.org/10.1016/j.jaci.2013.07.049. Epub 2013 Oct 24.
3. Deleuran MS, Vestergaard C. Therapy of severe atopic dermatitis in adults. J Dtsch Dermatol Ges. 2012;10(6):399–406. https://doi.org/10.1111/j.1610-0387.2012.07899_suppl.x.
4. Russell G, Graveley R, Seid J, Al-Humidan A-K, Skjodt H. Mechanisms of action of cyclosporine and effects on connective tissues. Semin Arthritis Rheum. 1992;21(6):16–22. https://doi.org/10.1016/0049-0172(92)90009-3.
5. van Joost T, Heule F, Korstanje M, van den Broek MJ, Stenveld HJ, van Vloten WA. Cyclosporin in atopic dermatitis: a multicentre placebo-controlled study. Br J Dermatol. 1994;130(5):634–40. https://doi.org/10.1111/j.1365-2133.1994.tb13111.x.
6. Brunner PM, Guttman-Yassky E, Leung DY. The immunology of atopic dermatitis and its reversibility with broad-spectrum and targeted therapies. J Allergy Clin Immunol. 2017;139(4S):S65–76. https://doi.org/10.1016/j.jaci.2017.01.011.
7. Schmitt J, Schäkel K, Fölster-Holst R, Bauer A, Oertel R, Augustin M, Aberer W, Luger T, Meurer M. Prednisolone vs. ciclosporin for severe adult eczema. An investigator-initiated double-blind placebo-controlled multicentre trial. Br J Dermatol. 2010;162(3):661–8. https://doi.org/10.1111/j.1365-2133.2009.09561.x. Epub 2009 Oct 26.
8. Schmitt J, Schmitt N, Meurer M. Cyclosporin in the treatment of patients with atopic eczema—a systematic review and meta-analysis. J Eur Acad Dermatol Venereol. 2007;21:606–19. https://doi.org/10.1111/j.1468-3083.2006.02023.x.
9. Berth-Jones J, Exton LS, Ladoyanni E, Mohd Mustapa MF, Tebbs VM, Yesudian PD, Levell NJ. British Association of Dermatologists guidelines for the safe and effective prescribing of oral ciclosporin in dermatology 2018. Br J Dermatol. 2019;180(6):1312–38. https://doi.org/10.1111/bjd.17587. Epub 2019 Apr 7.
10. Gooderham M, Lynde CW, Papp K, Bourcier M, Guenther L, Gulliver W, Hong CH, Poulin Y, Sussman G, Vender R. Review of systemic treatment options for adult atopic dermatitis. J Cutan Med Surg. 2017;21(1):31–9. https://doi.org/10.1177/1203475416670364. Epub 2016 Sep 22.
11. Mistry N, Gupta A, Alavi A, Sibbald RG. A review of the diagnosis and management of erythroderma (generalized red skin). Adv Skin Wound Care. 2015;28(5):228–36; quiz 237–8. https://doi.org/10.1097/01.ASW.0000463573.40637.73.
12. Megna M, Napolitano M, Patruno C, Villani A, Balato A, Monfrecola G, Ayala F, Balato N. Systemic treatment of adult atopic dermatitis: a review. Dermatol Ther (Heidelb). 2017;7(1):1–23. https://doi.org/10.1007/s13555-016-0170-1. Epub 2016 Dec 26.
13. Sekhon S, Bhutani T, Koo JYM. 17—Cyclosporine. In: Wolverton SE, editor. Comprehensive dermatologic drug therapy. 4th ed. Elsevier; 2021. p. 187–198.e3.
14. Davari DR, Nieman EL, McShane DB, Morrell DS. Current perspectives on the systemic management of atopic dermatitis. J Asthma Allergy. 2021;14:595–607. https://doi.org/10.2147/JAA.S287638.
15. Berth-Jones J, Voorhees JJ. Consensus conference on cyclosporin A microemulsion for psoriasis, June 1996. Br J Dermatol. 1996;135(5):775–7. https://doi.org/10.1046/j.1365-2133.1996.d01-1061.x. PMID: 8977680.
16. Ludwig CM, Krase JM, Price KN, Lio PA, Shi VY. A practical guide for transitioning from classical immunosuppressants to dupilumab in atopic dermatitis. J Dermatol Treat. 2021;32(5):503–6. https://doi.org/10.1080/09546634.2019.1682498. Epub 2019 Nov 25.

17. Paul CF, Ho VC, McGeown C, Christophers E, Schmidtmann B, Guillaume JC, Lamarque V, Dubertret L. Risk of malignancies in psoriasis patients treated with cyclosporine: a 5 years cohort study. J Invest Dermatol. 2003;120(2):211–6. https://doi.org/10.1046/j.1523-1747.2003.12040.x.
18. Mrowietz U, de Jong EM, Kragballe K, Langley R, Nast A, Puig L, Reich K, Schmitt J, Warren RB. A consensus report on appropriate treatment optimization and transitioning in the management of moderate-to-severe plaque psoriasis. Journal of the european academy of dermatology and venereology: JEADV. 2014;28(4):438–53. https://doi.org/10.1111/jdv.12118.

# Chapter 14
# Treatment of AD with Tralokinumab

**Kareem G. Elhage, Riley K. Spencer, Joy Q. Jin, Mitchell S. Davis, Marwa Hakimi, Tina Bhutani, and Wilson Liao**

**Case Title** A 28-year-old male with long-standing atopic dermatitis presents with acute onset of a unilateral, vesicular rash

### Case

A 28-year-old male patient with a long-standing history of severe atopic dermatitis (AD) presents to your dermatology clinic with a painful rash on his back. Initially, he tried managing his AD with topical medications and phototherapy, but after both failed to improve his condition, he was prescribed abrocitinib 2 months ago. He mentions that before he noticed the new painful rash, he had been experiencing pain and tingling in the same region. He has also felt generally unwell, endorsing sensitivity to light and a headache. On physical exam, you observe a unilateral rash that wraps around the right side of his lower back. You also notice a cluster of vesicles. After considering the patient's symptoms, history, and physical exam, a clinical diagnosis is made.

### Board Review Question

After discussing with the patient, you decide to switch him to another medication for his AD. Of the following options, which is the best management option?

K. G. Elhage · R. K. Spencer · M. S. Davis · M. Hakimi · T. Bhutani · W. Liao (✉)
Department of Dermatology, University of California at San Francisco,
San Francisco, CA, USA
e-mail: kareem.elhage@ucsf.edu; Riley.Spencer@ucsf.edu; Mitchell.Davis@ucsf.edu; Tina.Bhutani@ucsf.edu; wilson.liao@ucsf.edu

J. Q. Jin
Department of Dermatology, University of California at San Francisco,
San Francisco, CA, USA

School of Medicine, University of California at San Francisco, San Francisco, CA, USA
e-mail: Joy.Jin@ucsf.edu



N. Brownstone et al. (eds.), *Clinical Cases in Atopic Dermatitis*, Clinical Cases in Dermatology, https://doi.org/10.1007/978-3-031-52147-8_14

A. Upadacitinib
B. Tralokinumab
C. Topical tacrolimus
D. Baricitinib
E. Triamcinolone

## Main Text

Atopic dermatitis (AD) is a chronic, inflammatory skin disease characterized by severe pruritus and eczematous lesions. With an estimated prevalence of 2.1–4.9% in North America, AD represents significant disease burden among patients [1]. Furthermore, the disease is associated with significant pain, sleep disruption, and mental health conditions, including anxiety and depression. To address the disease and its sequelae, efforts have been geared toward developing viable medications for the treatment of moderate-to-severe AD.

## Tralokinumab: Mechanism of Action

As researchers and physicians gain a better understanding of AD's pathogenesis and the inflammatory pathways that cause the disease, treatments may target specific cytokines [2]. One of the cytokines involved in AD's pathogenesis is IL-13, which is a type 2 cytokine implicated in several factors that contribute to the disease severity, including skin barrier disruption, inflammation, itch, and increased risk of skin infection. Tralokinumab is a human monoclonal antibody that binds to IL-13, thereby preventing interaction with its receptor [3]. Various trials have shown its efficacy in providing long-term improvements in symptoms and disease signs of moderate-to-severe AD.

## Tralokinumab: Efficacy and Safety in Clinical Trials

ECZTRA 1 and ECZTRA 2 were the first phase III trials conducted to examine the safety and efficacy of tralokinumab in the treatment of moderate-to-severe AD [1]. Both trials consisted of randomized, double-blind, placebo-controlled trials that were conducted over the course of 52 weeks, with 802 and 794 patients enrolled, respectively. Patients were randomized to either placebo or subcutaneous tralokinumab at a loading dose of 600 mg followed by 300 mg every other week. To analyze treatment outcomes, an Investigator's Global Assessment (IGA) score of 0 (clear skin) or 1 (almost clear skin) and the Eczema Area and Severity Index (EASI) 75 (indicates 75% improvement of EASI score from baseline) were used as primary endpoints. Secondary endpoints included daily pruritus numerical rating score (NRS), SCORing Atopic Dermatitis (SCORAD), and the Dermatology Life Quality Index (DLQI) (Table 14.1).

At the end of the initial 16-week evaluation period in both studies, patients in the tralokinumab group were significantly more likely to achieve an IGA score of 0 or 1 and EASI 75 than patients in the placebo group. Furthermore, in ECZTRA 1, 15.8% of patients in the tralokinumab group achieved an IGA score of 0 or 1, while only 7.1% of patients in the placebo group achieved the same endpoint. ECZTRA 2 displayed similar results, with 22.2% of patients in the tralokinumab group vs 10.9% in the placebo group achieving an IGA of 0 or 1.

Regarding EASI 75, in ECZTRA 1, 25% of patients in the tralokinumab group versus 12.7% of patients in the placebo group achieved this endpoint. In ECZTRA 2, 33.2% of patients in the tralokinumab group versus 11.4% of patients in the placebo group reached EASI 75. In both trials, these differences were found to be statistically significant. Furthermore, changes in daily pruritus NRS, SCORAD, and DLQI were all found to be significantly different, with patients in the tralokinumab group consistently achieving better outcomes than their placebo group counterparts.

ECZTRA 3, another double-blind, randomized, placebo-controlled trial, was conducted over the course of 32 weeks and evaluated the use of tralokinumab in combination with topical corticosteroids (TCS) as needed versus placebo with TCS as needed [4]. Three hundred eighty patients were enrolled in the study. Similar to ECZTRA 1 and 2, primary endpoints included achieving an IGA of 0 or 1 and EASI 75 at week 16, while secondary endpoints were comprised of improvements in pruritus NRS, SCORAD, and DLQI. At the end of the trial period, significantly more patients in the tralokinumab and TCS group achieved the primary endpoints than patients in the placebo and TCS group: 38.9% and 56% of patients in the tralokinumab and TCS group versus 26.2% and 35.7% of patients in the placebo and TCS group achieved an IGA of 0 or 1 and EASI 75, respectively. Furthermore, patients in the tralokinumab group were significantly more likely to achieve all secondary endpoints than their placebo group counterparts.

**Table 14.1** Characteristics of included phase III randomized, placebo-controlled trials

| | ECZTRA 1 [1] | | ECZTRA 2 [1] | | ECZTRA 3 [5] | |
|---|---|---|---|---|---|---|
| | Tralokinumab Q2W (*N* = 603) | Placebo (*N* = 199) | Tralokinumab Q2W (*N* = 593) | Placebo (*N* = 201) | Tralokinumab Q2W + TCS (*N* = 253) | Placebo + TCS (*N* = 127) |
| Age (median (IQR)) | 37.0 (27.0–48.0) | 37.0 (26.0–49.0) | 34.0 (25.0–48.0) | 30.0 (23.0–46.0) | 37.0 (28.0–52.0) | 34.0 (24.0–50.0) |
| Sex (*N* (%)) | | | | | | |
| Male | 351 (58.2%) | 123 (61.8%) | 359 (60.5%) | 114 (56.7%) | 125 (49.4%) | 84 (66.1%) |
| Female | 252 (41.8%) | 76 (38.2%) | 234 (39.5%) | 87 (43.3%) | 128 (50.8%) | 43 (33.9%) |
| Race (*N* (%)) | | | | | | |
| White | 426 (70.6%) | 138 (69.3%) | 374 (63.1%) | 123 (61.2%) | 203 (80.2%) | 85 (66.9%) |
| Black or African American | 41 (6.8%) | 18 (9.0%) | 43 (7.3%) | 17 (8.5%) | 23 (9.1%) | 12 (9.4%) |
| Asian | 120 (19.9%) | 41 (20.1%) | 154 (26.0%) | 52 (25.9%) | 17 (6.7%) | 24 (18.9%) |
| Native Hawaiian or other Pacific islander | – | – | – | – | 1 (0.4%) | 1 (0.8%) |
| Other | 16 (2.6%) | 3 (1.5%) | 22 (3.7%) | 9 (4.5%) | 9 (3.6%) | 5 (3.9%) |
| % BSA affected (median (IQR)) | 50.0% (33.0–70.0%) | 52.5% (31.0–77.0%) | 50.0% (31.0–74.0%) | 50.0% (31.0–74.0%) | 41.0% (30.0–63.0%) | 40.0% (26.0–74.0%) |
| Severe AD/IGA score of 4 (N (%)) | 305 (50.6%) | 102 (51.3%) | 286 (48.2%) | 101 (50.2%) | 116 (45.8%) | 60 (47.2%) |
| EASI score (median (IQR)) | 28.2 (21.3–40.0) | 30.3 (22.0–41.5) | 28.2 (19.8–40.8) | 29.6 (20.6–41.4) | 24.7 (18.4–35.9) | 26.5 (19.9–39.3) |

| | | | | | | |
|---|---|---|---|---|---|---|
| DLQI score (median (IQR)) | 17.0 (12.0–22.0) | 16.0 (13.0–22.0) | 18.0 (13.0–23.0) | 18.0 (12.5–24.0) | 18.0 (12.0–23.0) | 18.0 (12.0–23.) |
| Pruritus NRS (median (IQR)) | 7.9 (6.7–8.9) | 7.9 (6.9–8.7) | 8.0 (7.0–9.0) | 8.1 (7.1–9.0) | 8.0 (6.6–8.7) | 8.0 (7.0–9.0) |
| SCORAD (median (IQR)) | 69.2 (61.5–79.1) | 70.8 (63.8–81.0) | 69.5 (60.5–79.1) | 69.9 (61.9–79.1) | 66.2 (57.6–76.3) | 67.9 (59.4–79.0) |

This table includes study design, demographics, primary endpoints, and secondary endpoints for tralokinumab and placebo groups in clinical trials ECZTRA 1 (NCT03131648), ECZTRA 2 (NCT03160885), and ECZTRA 3 (NCT03363854)

*AD* Atopic dermatitis, *BSA* Body surface area involvement, *DLQI* Dermatology Life Quality Index, *EASI* Eczema Area and Severity Index, *IGA* Investigator's Global Assessment, *IQR* Interquartile range, *NRS* Numeric Rating Scale, *Q2W* Every 2 weeks, *SCORAD* SCORing Atopic Dermatitis, *TCS* Topical corticosteroids

## Tralokinumab: Safety Considerations

To assess the safety of tralokinumab, a pooled analysis of five randomized, double-blind, placebo-controlled phase II and III trials was conducted [5]. The analysis included the three aforementioned phase III studies (ECZTRA 1, ECZTRA 2, and ECZTRA 3), one-phase IIb dose-finding trial, and one-phase II vaccine response trial (ECZTRA 5). A total of 680 patients included in the pooled analysis were part of a placebo group, while 1605 received tralokinumab. The frequency of any adverse event (AE) was 65.7% in the tralokinumab group and 67.2% in the placebo group. Of these reported AEs, 4.6% and 6.3% were considered severe in the tralokinumab and placebo groups, respectively. Only 2.3% and 2.8% of events lead to permanent discontinuation of study drug in the tralokinumab and placebo groups, respectively.

In both groups, AD flares were the most commonly encountered AE. Other common AEs included viral upper respiratory tract infection, conjunctivitis, upper respiratory tract infection, and injection site reaction, all of which occurred more frequently in patients receiving tralokinumab than those receiving placebo. Notably, skin infections occurred at lower rates in patients taking tralokinumab than those receiving placebo. Additionally, 2.1% and 2.8% of patients in the tralokinumab and placebo groups experienced serious adverse events (SAE), respectively, with infection and infestation being the most commonly reported SAEs. However, less than 1% of patients experienced an SAE that led to permanent study drug discontinuation. There were no safety concerns regarding the development of herpes zoster in patients taking tralokinumab, which was a concern in clinical trials of Janus kinase (JAK) inhibitors [6, 7].

IL-13 has been shown to play a key role in driving inflammation in AD [3]. Dupilumab, a drug that blocks both IL-4 and IL-13, was previously the only approved biologic for the treatment of moderate-to-severe AD. However, tralokinumab—a human immunoglobulin that binds to IL-13 and prevents its downstream signaling—has shown promise in a number of phase III clinical trials. In all of the aforementioned clinical trials, patients receiving tralokinumab achieved both primary and secondary endpoints across both physical and psychological domains at significantly higher rates than those receiving placebo or TCS. Furthermore, patients receiving tralokinumab were not at a significantly higher risk of experiencing AEs or SAEs, which highlights its safety. Thus, tralokinumab represents a safe and effective treatment modality for moderate-to-severe AD.

**Board Review Question Explanation**

After discussing with the patient, you decide to switch him to another medication for his AD. Of the following options, which is the best management option?

A. Upadacitinib
B. Tralokinumab (correct)
C. Topical tacrolimus
D. Baricitinib
E. Triamcinolone

**Explanation**

The correct answer is B (tralokinumab). The patient's prodromal symptoms of general malaise, pain, tingling, and physical findings of a unilateral, vesicular rash in the setting of long-standing, severe AD treated with abrocitinib are characteristic of herpes zoster. A wide variety of therapies are available for AD, including topical corticosteroids (triamcinolone), tacrolimus, JAK inhibitors (abrocitinib, upadacitinib), and biologics (dupilumab, tralokinumab). Studies have shown that patients receiving abrocitinib are at greater risk of developing herpes zoster. Conversely, studies have shown no concerns over the safety of tralokinumab regarding the development of herpes zoster.

**References:**

- Blauvelt A, Teixeira HD, Simpson EL, et al. Efficacy and safety of upadacitinib vs dupilumab in adults with moderate-to-severe atopic dermatitis: a randomized clinical trial. JAMA Dermatol 2021;157(9):1047–55. doi:10.1001/jamadermatol.2021.3023.
- Simpson EL, Merola JF, Silverberg JI, et al. Safety of tralokinumab in adult patients with moderate-to-severe atopic dermatitis: pooled analysis of five randomized, double-blind, placebo-controlled phase II and phase III trials. Br J Dermatol 2022;187 (6):888–99. doi:10.1111/bjd.21867.

**Key Takeaway Points**

- Tralokinumab is a human monoclonal antibody that prevents IL-13 from interacting with its receptor, thereby decreasing inflammation in atopic dermatitis.
- Prior to the introduction of tralokinumab, dupilumab was the only biologic approved for the treatment of moderate-to-severe AD.
- Tralokinumab has demonstrated safety and efficacy as a treatment for moderate-to-severe AD in several randomized, placebo-controlled clinical trials.
- Both physical and psychological symptoms associated with AD significantly improved after treatment with tralokinumab when compared to placebo groups.
- When compared to other medications commonly used for the treatment of moderate-to-severe AD—such as JAK inhibitors—tralokinumab showed no safety concerns regarding the development of herpes zoster.

## References

1. Wollenberg A, Blauvelt A, Guttman-Yassky E, et al. Tralokinumab for moderate-to-severe atopic dermatitis: results from two 52-week, randomized, double-blind, multicentre, placebo-controlled phase III trials (ECZTRA 1 and ECZTRA 2). Br J Dermatol. 2021;184(3):437–49. https://doi.org/10.1111/bjd.19574.
2. Wollenberg A, Barbarot S, Bieber T, et al. Consensus-based European guidelines for treatment of atopic eczema (atopic dermatitis) in adults and children: part II. J Eur Acad Dermatol Venereol. 2018;32(6):850–78. https://doi.org/10.1111/jdv.14888.

3. Popovic B, Breed J, Rees DG, et al. Structural characterisation reveals mechanism of IL-13-neutralising monoclonal antibody tralokinumab as inhibition of binding to IL-13Rα1 and IL-13Rα2. J Mol Biol. 2017;429(2):208–19. https://doi.org/10.1016/j.jmb.2016.12.005.
4. Silverberg JI, Toth D, Bieber T, et al. Tralokinumab plus topical corticosteroids for the treatment of moderate-to-severe atopic dermatitis: results from the double-blind, randomized, multicentre, placebo-controlled phase III ECZTRA 3 trial. Br J Dermatol. 2021;184(3):450–63. https://doi.org/10.1111/bjd.19573.
5. Simpson EL, Merola JF, Silverberg JI, et al. Safety of tralokinumab in adult patients with moderate-to-severe atopic dermatitis: pooled analysis of five randomized, double-blind, placebo-controlled phase II and phase III trials. Br J Dermatol. 2022;187(6):888–99. https://doi.org/10.1111/bjd.21867.
6. Gooderham MJ, Forman SB, Bissonnette R, et al. Efficacy and safety of oral janus kinase 1 inhibitor abrocitinib for patients with atopic dermatitis: a phase 2 randomized clinical trial. JAMA Dermatol. 2019;155(12):1371–9. https://doi.org/10.1001/jamadermatol.2019.2855.
7. Silverberg JI, Simpson EL, Thyssen JP, et al. Efficacy and safety of abrocitinib in patients with moderate-to-severe atopic dermatitis: a randomized clinical trial. JAMA Dermatol. 2020;156(8):863–73. https://doi.org/10.1001/jamadermatol.2020.1406.

# Chapter 15
# Treatment of AD with Abrocitinib

**Joy Q. Jin, Riley K. Spencer, Kareem G. Elhage, Mitchell S. Davis, Marwa Hakimi, Wilson Liao, and Tina Bhutani**

**Case Title** A 34-year-old male with eczematous patches and plaques involving the neck, torso, and extremities who discontinued dupilumab due to side effects

**Case**
A 34-year-old male with childhood-onset atopic dermatitis, allergies, and asthma presents for a follow-up visit. He was diagnosed as a toddler with eczema and has sporadically seen a dermatologist for skin flares. Today, he presents with another flare that he feels is itchier and more impactful to his quality of life, which has been progressively worsening over the past 2 years. His previous dermatologist prescribed him a course of dupilumab, but this was discontinued as he experienced extremely itchy and irritated eyes after using the medication for 6 months. He currently uses two over-the-counter moisturizers that he applies daily, as well as some leftover topical steroids (currently clobetasol propionate cream, 0.05%) that he applies twice a day.

He self-reports that his current symptoms are not well-controlled, as he experiences 7/10 itch and the eczema is currently affecting his sleep quality. He mentions that if he were to explore another systemic medication option for his AD, he would

J. Q. Jin
School of Medicine, University of California at San Francisco, San Francisco, CA, USA

Department of Dermatology, University of California at San Francisco,
San Francisco, CA, USA
e-mail: joy.jin@ucsf.edu

R. K. Spencer · K. G. Elhage · M. S. Davis · M. Hakimi · W. Liao · T. Bhutani (✉)
Department of Dermatology, University of California at San Francisco,
San Francisco, CA, USA
e-mail: Riley.Spencer@ucsf.edu; kareem.elhage@med.wayne.edu; Mitchell.Davis@ucsf.edu; wilson.liao@ucsf.edu; Tina.Bhutani@ucsf.edu



N. Brownstone et al. (eds.), *Clinical Cases in Atopic Dermatitis*, Clinical Cases in Dermatology, https://doi.org/10.1007/978-3-031-52147-8_15

prefer an oral therapy as he is worried about injecting himself with a needle after his experience using dupilumab. On exam, he exhibits ill-defined, erythematous patches and lichenified plaques with overlying excoriations on the neck, abdomen, back, and extremities—including flexural areas and forearms—covering about 10% of his body surface area. What treatment option would you recommend for this patient?

**Board Review Question**

What three laboratory tests should be ordered before initiating an AD patient on abrocitinib?

A. Complete blood count, tuberculosis test, and hepatitis B/C screening
B. Complete blood count, thyroid panel, and tuberculosis test
C. Tuberculosis test, thyroid panel, and hepatitis B/C screening
D. Complete blood count, tuberculosis test, and C-reactive protein level
E. Tuberculosis test, urinalysis, and hepatitis B/C screening

## Main Text

Atopic dermatitis (AD) management is informed by disease severity, which includes extent of body surface area (BSA) involvement and impact of pruritus, as well as medical comorbidities and patient goals. The mainstays of treatment include emollients and topical therapies such as corticosteroids or calcineurin inhibitors. In moderate-to-severe AD, which affects up to 30% of patients, systemic therapy is often utilized and provides significant improvements to quality of life [1, 2]. Dupilumab is a popular biologic option that targets interleukin (IL)-4 and IL13—while dupilumab efficacy is often superior to alternatives, non-response is not infrequent and has been reported in up to 50% of AD patients in some previously published cohort studies [3]. Furthermore, some patients may experience poor efficacy of the drug following an initial period of clinical response—other individuals may prefer oral systemic medications due to ease of use, experience side effects that require them to switch to an alternative drug, or experience non-medical drug failure (e.g., due to insurance changes). In such cases, a systemic oral option such as abrocitinib, a Janus kinase (JAK) inhibitor, may be preferable. In this chapter, we will discuss the treatment of AD with abrocitinib, including a review of the medication's mechanism of action, treatment considerations, clinical trial data encompassing safety and efficacy, and lab monitoring requirements.

## Abrocitinib: Mechanism of Action

JAK inhibitors, such as abrocitinib, target intracellular JAK enzymes that mediate inflammatory signaling dysregulated in AD [4]. There are four members of the JAK family, including JAK1, JAK2, JAK3, and tyrosine kinase (TYK) 2. JAKs are activated following extracellular ligand (e.g., interleukins) binding to cell-membrane receptors, causing receptor dimerization—bringing the intracellular components of the dimerized receptors closer together such that JAKs can trans-phosphorylate each other and activate subsequent intracellular signaling [5]. Activated JAKs can phosphorylate STAT molecules; once activated, STAT then dissociates from the receptor to translocate to the nucleus, serving as a transcription factor [6].

In AD, JAK/STAT signaling can be activated by IL-4, which regulates T helper 2 (Th2) cell differentiation [6]. Upregulation of the Th2 immune response through JAK/STAT signaling causes hypersecretion of cytokines, chemokines, angiogenic factors, and IgE production—all of which exacerbate the AD inflammatory cycle [6]. Furthermore, upregulated JAK/STAT signaling may lead to breakdown in the natural skin barrier through stimulation of interferon (IFN)-$\gamma$ and IL-31, compounding the risk of AD flares and secondary complications such as infection [6]. As a result, therapeutics that inhibit the overactive components of JAK/STAT signaling may provide targeted relief in AD, which exhibits Th2-predominant pathogenesis.

Currently, two systemic JAK inhibitors are approved for the treatment of AD in the United States (US): abrocitinib (Cibinqo) and upadacitinib (Rinvoq). Other JAK inhibitors include baricitinib (Olumiant)—approved for AD treatment in the European Union but not in the US at the time of writing—and gusacitinib, which is currently under Food and Drug Administration (FDA) Fast Track investigation for the treatment of hand eczema. Abrocitinib and upadacitinib are selective JAK1 inhibitors that have significantly reduced affinity for other members of the JAK family [7]. As JAK2, JAK3, and TYK2 have been reported to influence hematopoietic stem cell lineages, lymphocyte development, and other immune cell differentiation processes, reduced affinity for these members has the potential to reduce the risk of unwanted complications such as anemia and thromboembolic events [7].

## Abrocitinib: Efficacy and Safety in Clinical Trials

The efficacy and safety of abrocitinib were examined in one phase IIB (NCT02780167) and six phase III (JADE MONO-1 NCT03349060, JADE MONO-2 NCT03575871, JADE REGIMEN NCT03627767, JADE COMPARE NCT03720470, JADE TEEN NCT03796676, JADE DARE NCT04345367) clinical trials, carried out between 2016 and 2021 [7].

The phase IIB trial examined a primary endpoint of Investigator's Global Assessment (IGA) and secondary endpoints including Eczema Area Severity Index (EASI) and quality of life, all measured at week 12 of abrocitinib treatment. Short-term use of abrocitinib at both 100 and 200 mg was found to significantly improve these endpoints compared to placebo use in patients with moderate-to-severe AD. Subsequent phase III trials also found significant improvements in IGA (e.g., percentage of patients achieving IGA of 0/1), EASI (e.g., patients achieving 75% clearance of AD as measured by EASI), and pruritus in both adolescent (12 through

17 years old) and adult (18+) age groups using various abrocitinib dosing regimens in comparison to placebo [7, 8]. For instance, JADE COMPARE NCT03720470 found that 36.6% and 48.4% of patients who received 100 mg abrocitinib and 200 mg abrocitinib, respectively, achieved an IGA of clear or almost clear AD by week 12 of treatment [7]. JADE DARE NCT04345367, which compared abrocitinib 200 mg once daily to the standard dupilumab dosing regimen at 300 mg every 2 weeks, found more patients on abrocitinib achieved improvements in pruritus at weeks 2 and 4 following treatment, as well as EASI 90 at week 16, suggesting that abrocitinib may have the potential to improve disease severity and itch to a greater degree than dupilumab [7].

Adverse events reported in clinical trials are summarized in Table 15.1. Most published clinical trials compared abrocitinib to placebo use and, on average, found slightly increased frequencies of short-term adverse events (AEs) developing in patients who were taking the highest dose of abrocitinib [7]. On average, AEs occurred at a frequency of 68.3%, 61.0%, and 55.0% in patient cohorts receiving abrocitinib 200 mg, abrocitinib 100 mg, and placebo, respectively [9]. Up to 94.2% of AEs were mild and self-limited and did not preclude continued use of abrocitinib. The most commonly reported AEs were nausea, nasopharyngitis, headache, upper respiratory tract infection, acne, vomiting, dizziness, herpes simplex, diarrhea, urinary tract infection, and folliculitis [7]. When comparing abrocitinib use at 200 mg and 100 mg doses, similar proportions of long-term and serious AEs occurred in both groups. In general, serious AEs were rare (3.8% and 5.4% in the 200 mg and 100 mg dosing groups) and included serious infections, herpes simplex, herpes zoster, eczema herpeticum, malignancy, major adverse cardiovascular events (MACEs), venous thromboembolism (VTE), and transient ischemic attack (TIA) [7]. Notably, conjunctivitis was not commonly reported in abrocitinib clinical trials, which contrasts with one of the most commonly reported side effects of dupilumab use, allowing abrocitinib to serve as an alternate systemic option for patients who cannot tolerate dupilumab, as seen in the patient case proposed in this chapter [7]. Finally, a recent network meta-analysis found no statistically significant risk difference of AE occurrence between abrocitinib, baricitinib, upadacitinib, and dupilumab—although results should be interpreted with caution given limitations in follow-up data (up to 40 weeks) and between-study heterogeneity [10].

## Abrocitinib: Treatment and Monitoring Recommendations

Abrocitinib was FDA-approved in early 2022 for the treatment of moderate-to-severe AD in individuals 18 years old or up who have experienced inadequate response to other systemic medications or when such options are contraindicated [7] (Table 15.1). Notably, upadacitinib is approved for individuals over the age of 12 [7]. Abrocitinib is not recommended if the patient is currently using other JAK inhibitors, biologic immunomodulators, or immunosuppressants [11]. There is currently limited data on abrocitinib use in individuals who are pregnant or

**Table 15.1** Abrocitinib contraindications, screening and monitoring considerations, and reported adverse events for atopic dermatitis treatment

| Contraindications | Screening labs | Lab monitoring | Adverse events |
|---|---|---|---|
| • Severe renal or hepatic impairment<br>• Individuals who are currently pregnant or breastfeeding<br>• Co-administration of drugs that inhibit or strongly induce CYP2C19 and CYP2C9<br>• Co-administration of drugs that are P-gp substrates (e.g., digoxin)<br>• Co-administration of anti-platelet therapy drugs (except aspirin 81 mg) during the first 3 months of treatment<br>• Co-administration with live vaccines given around the same time as abrocitinib initiation | • TB test (e.g., QuantiFERON gold)<br>• Hepatitis B and C screen<br>• CBC<br>Consider pregnancy evaluation, renal and hepatic evaluation, and dosage reduction in patients who are poor metabolizers of CYP2C19 or currently taking CYP2C19 inhibitors (e.g., fluvoxamine, fluconazole, probenecid) | • CBC: at baseline and at 4 weeks after initiation or dosage increase<br>• Lipid panel: at baseline and at 4 weeks after initiation | Listed in order of relative frequency based on published clinical trials (phase II, III, and extension studies):<br>• Nausea<br>• Headache<br>• Infection: nasopharyngitis, herpes simplex, herpes zoster<br>• Acne<br>• Vomiting<br>• Dizziness<br>• MACE<br>• Venous thromboembolism<br>• Transient ischemic attack |

*CBC* Complete blood count, *MACE* Major adverse cardiac event, *TB* Tuberculosis

breastfeeding; however, preliminary data of other JAK inhibitors such as tofacitinib studied for rheumatoid arthritis have found potential teratogenic effects in pregnant patients [8]. Thus, it is recommended that patients who are pregnant or lactating avoid abrocitinib use until further research studies yield more detailed findings.

The label for abrocitinib in the US does contain a black box warning for infection, mortality, malignancy, cardiovascular events, and thrombosis, similar to all other currently approved JAK inhibitors. A consensus statement published in 2020 by a 29-person committee involving multi-disciplinary physicians, providers, and patients found that JAK inhibitors may increase the risk of VTE, particularly in patients with a prior history of VTE, in rheumatoid arthritis [8]. A safety endpoint trial published in 2022 also noted a greater risk of major adverse cardiovascular events (MACE) and malignancy in rheumatoid arthritis patients greater than age 50 with at least one cardiovascular risk factor treated with tofacitinib, another oral JAK inhibitor, as compared to treatment with TNF-α inhibitors [12]. The literature surrounding AEs in AD is comparatively less robust; a systematic review published in 2021 found that data collected from 28 JAK inhibitor studies in AD was not suitable for meta-analysis given the relative lack of evidence for each individual JAK inhibitor and differences in patient eligibility criteria across the studies [13]. Given that the AD population tends to be younger in age with fewer comorbidities and concomitant medications than RA patients, the risk is likely reduced in this population. However, caution, risk-benefit analysis, and close monitoring should be discussed when treating older patients with cardiovascular risk factors; treatment with the lowest dose possible should be utilized.

The following tests should be performed prior to abrocitinib initiation: (1) Tuberculosis (TB) evaluation: in those with latent TB or at high risk for TB, a latent TB preventive regimen should be initiated prior to abrocitinib use. (2) Viral hepatitis B and C screening. (3) Complete blood count (CBC). Abrocitinib is not recommended if the patient exhibits the following: active TB, active hepatitis B or C, hepatic impairment, platelet count $<150{,}000/mm^3$, absolute lymphocyte count $<500/mm^3$, absolute neutrophil count $<1000/mm^3$, hemoglobin <8 g/dL, or began anti-platelet therapy within the last 3 months (excluding low-dose aspirin) [11].

Abrocitinib is available in 50, 100, and 200 mg oral tablets; the recommended starting dose is 100 mg once daily, taken with or without food [11]. Providers can consider increasing the dosage to a maximum of 200 mg per day if the starting dosage does not yield clinical efficacy following 12 weeks of administration [11]. Dosing should be adjusted for patients with renal impairment or if cytochrome inhibition (e.g., CYP2C19, CYP450) or metabolization is affected by concurrent medication use or patient genetics [11]. Once abrocitinib is begun, CBC evaluations are recommended at baseline, 4 weeks after treatment initiation, and 4 weeks after any dosage increase [11]. After 4 weeks of treatment, lipid monitoring is also recommended due to the risk of lipid elevation; providers may find that a lipid panel conducted at the time of abrocitinib initiation may be helpful to serve as a baseline for subsequent comparison [7]. Additional lab evaluations may be considered for patients on chronic abrocitinib who develop hematological abnormalities (e.g., reductions in platelet count, absolute lymphocyte count, absolute neutrophil count, or hemoglobin) [11]. Further considerations can be found on the manufacturer's medical information page [11].

**Board Review Question Explanation**

What three laboratory tests should be ordered before initiating an AD patient on abrocitinib?

A. Complete blood count, tuberculosis test, and hepatitis B/C screening (correct)
B. Complete blood count, thyroid panel, and tuberculosis test
C. Tuberculosis test, thyroid panel, and hepatitis B/C screening
D. Complete blood count, tuberculosis test, and C-reactive protein level
E. Tuberculosis test, urinalysis, and hepatitis B/C screening

**Explanation**

**Answer: A**. Three tests are recommended prior to abrocitinib initiation: (1) Tuberculosis (TB) evaluation: abrocitinib is contraindicated in those with active TB, and patients with latent TB or those at high risk for latent TB should begin TB treatment prior to abrocitinib use. (2) Viral hepatitis B and C screening: abrocitinib is contraindicated in patients with active hepatitis B or C. (3) Complete blood count (CBC): abrocitinib may cause decreases in white blood cells, platelets, or red blood cells, so baseline screening is recommended [11]. Additional tests that can be considered prior to abrocitinib use include a lipid panel screen, pregnancy test, basic metabolic panel to assess for renal function, and liver function tests depending on patient risk factors.

**Key Takeaway Points**

- Abrocitinib is an oral systemic medication taken once daily that targets Janus kinase (JAK) 1 signaling, inhibiting aberrant upregulation of T helper 2 (Th2)-mediated immune pathways involved in AD pathogenesis.
- Abrocitinib is approved for the use of moderate-to-severe AD in patients 18 years old and up and can serve as a good option for patients who have been failed by other systemic medications due to poor efficacy or side effects (e.g., conjunctivitis after dupilumab use).
- The most common adverse effects of abrocitinib include infections (ranging from nasopharyngitis to opportunistic infection), nausea, vomiting, and dizziness. There have been very few reported events of major adverse cardiac events and thrombosis.
- Prior to abrocitinib initiation, providers should screen for tuberculosis, hepatitis B and C, and hematologic abnormalities. While data in pregnant and breastfeeding individuals is limited, it is recommended to avoid JAK inhibitors such as abrocitinib until additional studies have been conducted.
- Once abrocitinib is initiated, providers should consider monitoring patients via a complete blood count and lipid panel at baseline and at 4 weeks after drug initiation or dosage increase, with additional monitoring considered on a case-by-case basis.

## References


1. Ständer S. Atopic Dermatitis. Ropper AH, editor. N Engl J Med [Internet]. 2021 Mar 25 [cited 2022 Dec 23];384(12):1136–43. https://pubmed.ncbi.nlm.nih.gov/33761208/
2. Lynde CW, Bourcier M, Gooderham M, Guenther L, Hong CH, Papp KA, et al. A treatment algorithm for moderate to severe Atopic dermatitis in adults. J Cutan Med Surg [Internet]. 2018;22(1):78–83. [cited 2022 Dec 23] Available from: https://pubmed.ncbi.nlm.nih.gov/29082775/
3. Linder C, Shourick J, Touhouche AT, Giordano-Labadie F, Severino-Freire M, Borjesson C, et al. Analysis of non-responders to dupilumab in clinical practice: a cohort study. J Eur Acad Dermatol Venereol [Internet]. 2021;35(3):e192–4. [cited 2022 Dec 23]. Available from: https://pubmed.ncbi.nlm.nih.gov/32870543/
4. Vazquez ML, Kaila N, Strohbach JW, Trzupek JD, Brown MF, Flanagan ME, et al. Identification of N-{cis-3-[methyl(7H-pyrrolo[2,3-d]pyrimidin-4-yl)amino]cyclobutyl} propane-1-sulfonamide (PF-04965842): a selective JAK1 clinical candidate for the treatment of autoimmune diseases. J Med Chem [Internet]. 2018;61(3):1130–52. [cited 2022 Dec 23]. Available from: https://pubmed.ncbi.nlm.nih.gov/29298069/
5. Chovatiya R, Paller AS. JAK inhibitors in the treatment of atopic dermatitis. J Allergy Clin Immunol [Internet]. 2021;148(4):927–40. [cited 2022 Dec 23]. Available from: https://pubmed.ncbi.nlm.nih.gov/34437922/
6. Szalus K, Trzeciak M, Nowicki RJ. JAK-STAT inhibitors in atopic dermatitis from pathogenesis to clinical trials results. Microorganisms [Internet]. 2020;8(11):1–14. [cited 2022 Dec 23]. Available from: /pmc/articles/PMC7694787/

7. Perche PO, Cook MK, Feldman SR. Abrocitinib: a new FDA-approved drug for moderate-to-severe atopic dermatitis. Ann Pharmacother [Internet]. 2022;57(1):86–98. [cited 2022 Dec 23]. https://doi-org.ucsf.idm.oclc.org/101177/10600280221096713. Available from: https://journals-sagepub-com.ucsf.idm.oclc.org/doi/10.1177/10600280221096713?url_ver=Z39.88-2003&rfr_id=ori%3Arid%3Acrossref.org&rfr_dat=cr_pub++0pubmed
8. Nash P, Kerschbaumer A, Dörner T, Dougados M, Fleischmann RM, Geissler K, et al. Points to consider for the treatment of immune-mediated inflammatory diseases with Janus kinase inhibitors: a consensus statement. Ann Rheum Dis [Internet]. 2021;80(1):71–87. [cited 2022 Dec 23]. Available from: https://pubmed.ncbi.nlm.nih.gov/33158881/
9. Simpson EL, Silverberg JI, Nosbaum A, Winthrop KL, Guttman-Yassky E, Hoffmeister KM, et al. Integrated safety analysis of abrocitinib for the treatment of moderate-to-severe atopic dermatitis from the phase II and phase III clinical trial program. Am J Clin Dermatol [Internet]. 2021;22(5):693–707. [cited 2022 Dec 23]. Available from: https://pubmed.ncbi.nlm.nih.gov/34406619/
10. Alves C, Penedones A, Mendes D, Batel MF. The safety of systemic Janus kinase inhibitors in atopic dermatitis: a systematic review and network meta-analysis. Eur J Clin Pharmacol [Internet]. 2022;78(12):1923–33. [cited 2022 Dec 23]. Available from: https://link.springer.com/article/10.1007/s00228-022-03400-4
11. CIBINQO Indications and Usage (abrocitinib) | Pfizer Medical Information—US [Internet]. [cited 2022 Dec 23]. https://www.pfizermedicalinformation.com/en-us/cibinqo-0/indications-usage
12. Ytterberg SR, Bhatt DL, Mikuls TR, Koch GG, Fleischmann R, Rivas JL, et al. Cardiovascular and cancer risk with tofacitinib in rheumatoid arthritis. N Engl J Med [Internet]. 2022;386(4):316–26. [cited 2023 Jan 10]. Available from: https://www.nejm.org/doi/full/10.1056/NEJMoa2109927
13. Le M, Berman-Rosa M, Ghazawi FM, Bourcier M, Fiorillo L, Gooderham M, et al. Systematic review on the efficacy and safety of oral janus kinase inhibitors for the treatment of atopic dermatitis. Front Med [Internet]. 2021;8:682547. [cited 2023 Jan 4]. Available from: /pmc/articles/PMC8440866/

# Chapter 16
# Treatment of AD with Upadacitinib

**Riley K. Spencer, Joy Q. Jin, Kareem G. Elhage, Mitchell S. Davis, Marwa Hakimi, Wilson Liao, and Tina Bhutani**

**Case Title** A 48-year-old female with a long-standing erythematous, lichenified, pruritic rash

**Case**
A new patient presents to your dermatology clinic, referred by a nearby primary care physician. She is a 48-year-old female and describes a 40-year history of an "itchy, red rash." She reports a constant struggle with intermittent flaring rashes since her teenage years but says the rash has looked "different" for the past decade. When she was younger, the rash would start as "itchy red bumps which oozed clear liquid when scratched" which would then crust over. Now, she describes her rash as "dark red, thick, and leathery from constant scratching," which always gets worse in the winter. She is unable to identify any alleviating factors, wears no jewelry, and has changed her shampoo, soap, and laundry detergent every 6 months to various fragrance-free options without any noticeable change in her skin condition. Her itch is rated as an 8/10 in severity, and she reports that her skin condition affects her

R. K. Spencer
Midwestern University, Arizona College of Osteopathic Medicine, Glendale, AZ, USA

University of California, San Francisco, CA, USA
e-mail: Riley.Spencer@ucsf.edu

J. Q. Jin
School of Medicine, University of California San Francisco, San Francisco, CA, USA
e-mail: Joy.Jin@ucsf.edu

K. G. Elhage
Wayne State University School of Medicine, Detroit, MI, USA
e-mail: kareem.elhage@med.wayne.edu

M. S. Davis · M. Hakimi · W. Liao · T. Bhutani (✉)
University of California, San Francisco, CA, USA
e-mail: Mitchell.Davis@ucsf.edu; wilson.liao@ucsf.edu; Tina.Bhutani@ucsf.edu



N. Brownstone et al. (eds.), *Clinical Cases in Atopic Dermatitis*, Clinical Cases in Dermatology, https://doi.org/10.1007/978-3-031-52147-8_16

quality of life in multiple areas including work productivity, sleep quality, self-confidence, and fashion choice.

Her current medication regimen includes clobetasol propionate 0.05% cream, triamcinolone 0.1% ointment, and fluocinonide 0.05% cream. Past medications include tacrolimus ointment, which was discontinued due to lack of efficacy, and cyclosporine which was discontinued to lab abnormalities. Her condition is complicated by poor medication adherence with topicals due to a "greasy feeling" and lack of skin improvement. The patient expresses frustration as cyclosporine was the only medication that really worked well for her, and she appreciated the convenience of an oral medication; however it was stopped due to elevated blood pressure readings and "something about her kidneys." She states that she is interested in pursuing new treatments. Her past medical history includes food allergies to peanuts, and family history includes asthma in her older brother and daughter.

Physical exam shows symmetric, poorly defined, erythematous patches and violaceous, lichenified plaques involving the volar forearms, popliteal creases, anterior neck, and trunk with an estimated body surface area involvement of 12%.

**Board Review Question**

Which of the following scenarios would make upadacitinib treatment for moderate-to-severe atopic dermatitis not advisable?

A. Active chronic obstructive pulmonary disease with daily administration of prophylactic low-dose erythromycin
B. Past medical history of multiple sclerosis
C. Recent skin biopsy showing spongiotic dermatitis, eosinophilic infiltrate, and intraepidermal vesicles
D. Last blood draw 2 months ago showing albumin 4.1 g/dL, INR 1.1, and total bilirubin of 0.9 mg/dL
E. History of Cushing's disease requiring daily administration of prednisone

## Main Text

Systemic immunomodulatory agents are indicated for patients with moderate-to-severe atopic dermatitis (AD) who fail topical or phototherapy regimens. Disease severity in AD is often stratified by validated, objective measurements like the Eczema Area and Severity Index (EASI) score, body surface area (BSA) percentage, and Investigator's Global Assessment (IGA) score, with an EASI $\geq$16, BSA $\geq$10%, and IGA $\geq$3 typically describing moderate-to-severe AD in clinical trials. Treatment decisions for these patients require integrating drug characteristics (efficacy, administration method, dosing schedule, potential side effects) with patient-specific factors (likelihood of adherence, comorbidities, contraindications).

For patients who require systemic agents to experience symptomatic relief and clinical improvement of their skin but prefer oral agents, several options are available. Older agents like cyclosporine, methotrexate, mycophenolate, and azathioprine may be highly effective and even produce rapid disease clearance in some cases. However, their utility in AD is limited due to the side effect profiles and contraindications associated with these drugs [1]. Janus kinase (JAK) inhibitors represent a novel class of systemic immunomodulatory agents which recently attained FDA approval for the treatment of refractory moderate-to-severe AD. These drugs inhibit the activity of JAK enzymes, with downstream effects on various inflammatory processes. Many of the cytokines implicated in the pathogenesis of atopic dermatitis mediate their effects via the JAK/STAT pathway. Upadacitinib and abrocitinib are JAK-1 specific inhibitors indicated for the treatment of moderate-to-severe AD. The following chapter reviews upadacitinib's mechanism of action, safety and efficacy data from clinical trials, comparative efficacy with alternative drugs, overall utility in AD, and lab monitoring recommendations.

## Mechanism of Action of JAK Inhibitors and Upadacitinib

Genome-wide studies implicate various cytokine signaling pathways as key mediators in many of the inflammatory processes in the pathogenesis of AD [2]. The inflammatory cascades involved in AD have been described as resulting from a biphasic T cell disease, with Th2 cytokines (interleukin (IL)-4, IL-13) dictating early stages of disease, with a switch to a Th1 response being seen in chronic AD [3]. This is evidenced by significantly increased expression of Th2 cytokines in lesional biopsies of acute AD and increased expression of Th1 cytokines (IFN-$\gamma$) in lesions of chronic AD [4]. Many of these cytokines, namely, IL-4, are dependent on JAKs, a family of non-receptor tyrosine kinases which phosphorylate and activate proteins in downstream signal transduction pathways. Type I and II cytokine receptor families possess no catalytic kinase activity, explaining their reliance on JAKs [5].

JAK/STAT signaling refers to a system consisting of three major components including (i) a dimeric, transmembrane cytokine receptor, (ii) a pair of intracellular JAKs, and (iii) a family of signal transducers and activators of transcription (STATs). The binding of cytokines to their respective receptors causes a conformational change in these dimeric proteins, leading to autophosphorylation of the intracellular JAKs, and another conformational change enabling phosphorylation of STATs. STATs then act as transcription factors, dissociating from the receptor complex and translocating to the nucleus to then regulate gene transcription [5].

The JAK family is comprised of four intracellular non-receptor tyrosine kinases, JAK1, JAK2, JAK3, and tyrosine kinase (TYK) 2. It has been proposed that the acute phase of AD mediated by Th2 cytokines primarily involves JAK1 and JAK3 activation via IL-4 signaling, while the Th1 lymphocyte signaling implicated in chronic AD may be mediated by JAK2 and TYK2 [6, 7]. Further, JAK/STAT signaling is thought to play a role in lymphocyte class-switching, production of IgE, and the epithelial barrier dysfunction inherent in AD [7]. Systemic immunomodulation in the form of JAK/STAT signaling inhibition has been shown to be an effective therapeutic option for AD, with two JAK-1 specific inhibitors, upadacitinib and abrocitinib, being FDA approved in the treatment of moderate-to-severe AD. Specifically, upadacitinib is an oral systemic agent providing targeted immunomodulation via a greater inhibitory potency for JAK1 versus other members in the JAK family.

## Clinical Trials Investigating Upadacitinib in AD

Measure Up 1 (NCT03569293) and Measure Up 2 (NCT03607422) were multicenter, double-blind, placebo-controlled phase 3 trials performed across Europe, North and South America, and Asia which investigated the use of upadacitinib in AD [8]. Both adolescent (12–17 years old) and adult (18–75 years old) patients with moderate to severe AD (≥10% BSA, EASI ≥16, validated IGA for Atopic Dermatitis [vIGA-AD] ≥3, and Worst Pruritus Numerical Rating Scale (NRS) ≥4) were included. Patients were randomized 1:1:1 to upadacitinib 15 mg, upadacitinib 30 mg, or placebo. Patients achieving a 75% improvement from baseline in the Eczema Area and Severity Index (EASI-75) at week 16 were significantly higher for both upadacitinib 15 mg (70%) and 30 mg (80%) groups versus placebo (16%) in Measure Up 1 [8]. This finding was reciprocated in Measure up 2 with 60% and 73% in the upadacitinib 15 mg and 30 mg groups, respectively, achieving EASI-75 response at week 16 versus 13% in the placebo group [8]. In both studies, the proportion of patients achieving a vIGA-AD response (vIGA-AD 0 or 1 with at least a 2-point improvement) was significantly higher in both upadacitinib groups as well.

In a head-to-head comparison of 924 patients with moderate to-severe atopic dermatitis (NCT03738397), upadacitinib 30 mg QD was superior to dupilumab 300 mg EOW in producing EASI-75 response at 16 weeks (71.0 vs. 61.1%) [9]. Upadacitinib also resulted in a greater rate of serious adverse events (SAEs) versus dupilumab (4.02% vs. 2.03%), including an increased incidence serious infection, eczema herpeticum, herpes zoster, and lab-related adverse events [9].

Network meta-analysis of seven phase IIb and III randomized clinical trials investigating upadacitinib and abrocitinib in atopic dermatitis assessed the comparative efficacy and safety profile of these two JAK-1 inhibitors. Statistical analysis demonstrated that upadacitinib was significantly superior to abrocitinib in producing both IGA 0 or 1 and EASI 75 responses [10]. Direct meta-analysis comparing the rates of treatment-emergent adverse events (TEAEs) demonstrated that both upadacitinib and abrocitinib had an increased incidence of TEAEs compared with placebo, while subgroup network meta-analysis showed that upadacitinib 30 mg was associated with a significantly increased incidence of TEAEs [10].

Adverse reactions (≥1%) reported in clinical trials of upadacitinib in atopic dermatitis include upper respiratory tract infections, cough, influenza, influenza-like illness, headache, fatigue, myalgia, abdominal pain, pyrexia, acne, folliculitis, herpes simplex, weight gain, neutropenia, and an increase in blood creatine phosphokinase levels [11].

## Treatment of AD with Upadacitinib and Lab Monitoring Recommendations

According to FDA recommendations, upadacitinib should be used only when a patient has had either an inadequate clinical response to another available systemic therapy or has contraindications to using these other agents. These other treatments include both traditional systemic agents (cyclosporine, methotrexate, mycophenolate, and azathioprine) and biologics (dupilumab, tralokinumab). While both upadacitinib and abrocitinib have received similar approval, key distinctions in their labels exist. Only upadacitinib is approved for both adults and adolescents (12 years and older, weighing at least 40 kg) [11], while abrocitinib is approved for use only in adults with moderate-to-severe atopic dermatitis [12]. It is recommended to initiate treatment with upadacitinib for atopic dermatitis starting with 15 mg orally QD, and if an adequate response is not achieved, consider an increase to 30 mg QD. Patients taking 30 mg with sustained disease remission may be considered for dose reduction. For adults 65 and older, and those with severe renal impairment, recommended dosing is 15 mg QD only [11].

Rinvoq, the marketed version of upadacitinib in the United States and Europe, carries a black box warning for serious infections. These reported infections included active tuberculosis (TB) (including extrapulmonary disease), invasive fungal infections (cryptococcosis, pneumocystosis), and bacterial, viral, and other opportunistic pathogenic organisms. However, concomitant immunosuppressants (corticosteroids, methotrexate, etc.) were being utilized in most patients who developed these infections, and use of upadacitinib in combination with other immunosuppressants is not recommended [11]. Patients being initiated on upadacitinib are recommended to be closely monitored for signs of infection and should have a negative TB test or be treated for latent TB prior to beginning treatment. It is recommended that upadacitinib be avoided in patients with active, serious infections (including localized infections) and those receiving live vaccines.

Upadacitinib also has a black box warning for all-cause mortality, malignancy, major adverse cardiovascular events (MACE), and thrombosis [11]. These recommendations are present on the labels for all JAK inhibitors and are based on the results of a safety endpoint trial showing a greater risk of these adverse events in rheumatoid arthritis patients older than age 50 with at least one cardiovascular risk factor being treated with tofacitinib, another oral JAK inhibitor, as compared to treatment with TNF-alpha inhibitors [13]. Given that the AD population tends to be younger, have less comorbidities, and less concomitant medications than RA patients, the risk is likely less for this population. However, caution, risk-benefit analysis, and close monitoring should be discussed when treating older patients with cardiovascular risk factors and treatment with the lowest dose possible should be utilized.

Considerations for special patient populations (pregnancy, lactation, etc.) can be found on the package insert or manufacturer's medical information page [11]. Pregnancy status of females of reproductive potential should be verified prior to initiating treatment with upadacitinib. Upadacitinib is a category D drug not recommended during pregnancy, with animal studies of upadacitinib demonstrating a potential for embryo-fetal harm during pregnancy [14]. Data on upadacitinib during lactation is unavailable and is thus not recommended during breastfeeding. Contraception while taking upadacitinib is advised for both males and females [15]. Upadacitinib is not recommended in patients with severe hepatic impairment (Child-Pugh C) [11]. Drug interactions have been reported with upadacitinib, and it is not recommended to administer upadacitinib alongside strong inducers of CYP3A4 (e.g., rifampin). For patients taking strong CYP3A4 inhibitors (e.g., ketoconazole), the recommended dosing of upadacitinib is 15 mg QD.

Counseling on the risk of serious hypersensitivity reactions (including anaphylaxis), and discontinuation should any such reaction occur, should be given to all patients initiated on upadacitinib. Patients at risk for gastrointestinal perforations should be monitored and promptly evaluated should they develop potential symptoms.

Given the contraindications and precautions associated with upadacitinib, appropriate pretreatment screening and risk assessment may be advisable. Aspects of patient medical history to consider include a history of venous thromboembolism, infections, tuberculosis, hepatitis B or C, cardiovascular disease, and concomitant medication use (e.g., CYP450 inducers/inhibitors, immunosuppressants). Assessment for non-melanoma skin cancers prior to initiating upadacitinib may be considered as well. Baseline lab monitoring prior to starting upadacitinib should include a TB evaluation (risk of TB reactivation with upadacitinib is similar to that of TNF-alpha inhibitors), viral hepatitis panel, complete blood count (CBC), liver enzymes, and lipid panel, unless recently performed [15]. Patients with evidence of chronic hepatitis B or hepatitis C infection should avoid treatment with upadacitinib. For those with risk factors for HIV infection, testing may be performed. Vaccination status may be investigated, and for patients requiring the administration of live-attenuated vaccines (e.g., herpes zoster), a 3- to 4-week postvaccination delay before initiating upadacitinib can be considered [15]. Patients taking upadacitinib who develop herpes zoster should pause upadacitinib until herpes zoster resolution.

Monitoring for laboratory abnormalities may be considered due to the potential for alterations in hematopoietic cell lines (lymphocytes, neutrophils, hemoglobin), liver enzymes, and lipid levels. Initiation of upadacitinib is not advisable in patients with an absolute lymphocyte or neutrophil counts (ALC, ANC) $<500$ cells/mm$^3$ or $<1000$ cells/mm$^3$, respectively. Lipid level alterations include an elevation of low-density lipoprotein (LDL) cholesterol and high-density lipoprotein (HDL) cholesterol with LDL levels decreasing to pre-treatments levels following statin therapy. Recommendations from Rinvoq's package insert and expert committees include liver enzymes and lipid parameter re-evaluation 12 weeks after the initiation of upadacitinib therapy and there-after according to routine patient management [11, 15]. Re-evaluation for neutropenia, lymphopenia, and anemia may be performed with a CBC according to routine patient management [11].

**Board Review Explanation**

Which of the following scenarios would make upadacitinib treatment for moderate-to-severe atopic dermatitis not advisable?

A. Active chronic obstructive pulmonary disease with daily administration of prophylactic low-dose erythromycin
B. Past medical history of multiple sclerosis
C. Recent skin biopsy showing spongiotic dermatitis, eosinophilic infiltrate, and intraepidermal vesicles
D. Last blood draw 2 months ago showing albumin 4.1 g/dL, INR 1.1, and total bilirubin of 0.9 mg/dL
E. History of Cushing's disease requiring daily administration of prednisone (correct)

**Explanation**

Rinvoq, the marketed version of upadacitinib, carries a black box warning for serious infections. This warning was issued based on infections developing primarily from patients being treated with upadacitinib and concomitant immunosuppressants (corticosteroids, methotrexate, etc.). As such, the combination of upadacitinib with other immunosuppressants is not recommended [11].

Erythromycin is a CYP3A4 inhibitor and will likely require dose adjustment of upadacitinib to a lower dose (e.g., 15 mg) but would not exclude upadacitinib treatment as an option.

A past medical history of multiple sclerosis, and other demyelinating diseases, is a contraindication to treatment with TNF-alpha inhibitors, not JAK-inhibitors. Further, TNF-alpha inhibitors are not FDA approved for the treatment of AD.

Accumulation of fluid leading to intercellular edema in the epidermis, also known as spongiosis, primarily characterizes the lesions of acute AD. Other findings include inflammatory infiltrate with eosinophils and intraepidermal vesicles. Conversely, marked thickening of the epidermis, termed acanthosis, and thickening of the stratum corneum layer (hyperkeratosis) are findings associated with chronic AD [16].

These lab values for albumin (3.4–5.4 g/dL), INR (1.1 and below), and bilirubin (0.1–1.2 mg/dL) are within reference ranges and do not indicate concern for hepatic insufficiency. Patients with evidence of severe liver disease on blood work (albumin <2.8 g/dL, INR >2.3 without concomitant warfarin administration, total bilirubin >3 mg/dL) or physical exam (abdominal fluid wave, asterixis, etc.) are poor candidates for upadacitinib treatment given its metabolism by the CYP-450 system.

**Key Takeaway Points**

- Upadacitinib is an oral, systemic, immunomodulating agent available in 15 or 30 mg formulations which selectively targets Janus kinase (JAK) 1 signaling pathways implicated in the pathogenesis of atopic dermatitis.
- Upadacitinib is approved for use in adolescent and adult patients with moderate-to-severe AD only when all other therapeutic options have been exhausted, due to either inadequate clinical response or contraindications.

- Rinvoq, the marketed version of upadacitinib in the United States and Europe, carries a black box warning for serious infections, mortality, malignancy, major adverse cardiovascular events (MACEs), and thrombosis.
- Baseline lab monitoring prior to starting upadacitinib should include a TB evaluation, viral hepatitis panel, complete blood count (CBC), liver enzymes, and lipid panel.

## References


1. Bußmann C, Novak N. Systemic therapy of atopic dermatitis. Allergol Select. 2017;1(1):1–8. https://doi.org/10.5414/ALX01285E.
2. Tamari M, Hirota T. Genome-wide association studies of atopic dermatitis. J Dermatol. 2014;41(3):213–20.
3. Gittler JK, et al. Progressive activation of T(H)2/T(H)22 cytokines and selective epidermal proteins characterizes acute and chronic atopic dermatitis. J Allergy Clin Immunol. 2012;130(6):1344–54.
4. Furue M, et al. Atopic dermatitis: immune deviation, barrier dysfunction, IgE autoreactivity and new therapies. Allergol Int. 2017;66(3):398–403.
5. Kisseleva, Bhattacharya S, Braunstein J, Schindler CW, et al. Signaling through the JAK/STAT pathway, recent advances and future challenges. Gene. 2002;285(1–2):1–24. https://doi.org/10.1016/S0378-1119(02)00398-0.
6. Howell MD, Kuo FI, Smith PA. Targeting the Janus kinase family in autoimmune skin diseases. Front Immunol. 2019;10:2342. https://doi.org/10.3389/fimmu.2019.02342.
7. Szalus K, Trzeciak M, Nowicki RJ. JAK-STAT inhibitors in atopic dermatitis from pathogenesis to clinical trials results. Microorganisms. 2020;8(11):1743. https://doi.org/10.3390/microorganisms8111743.
8. Guttman-Yassky E, Teixeira HD, Simpson EL, Papp KA, Pangan AL, Blauvelt A, Thaçi D, Chia-Yu Chu H, Hong C-h, Katoh N, Paller AS, Calimlim B, Yihua G, Xiaofei H, Liu M, Yang Y, Liu J, Tenorio AR, Chu AD, Irvine AD. Once-daily upadacitinib versus placebo in adolescents and adults with moderate-to-severe atopic dermatitis (Measure Up 1 and Measure Up 2): results from two replicate double-blind, randomised controlled phase 3 trials. Lancet. 2021;397(10290):2151–68, ISSN: 0140-6736. https://doi.org/10.1016/S0140-6736(21)00588-2.
9. Blauvelt A, Teixeira HD, Simpson EL, et al. Efficacy and safety of upadacitinib vs dupilumab in adults with moderate-to-severe atopic dermatitis: a randomized clinical trial. JAMA Dermatol. 2021;157(9):1047–55. https://doi.org/10.1001/jamadermatol.2021.3023.
10. Wan H, Jia H, Xia T, Zhang D. Comparative efficacy and safety of abrocitinib, baricitinib, and upadacitinib for moderate-to-severe atopic dermatitis: A network meta-analysis. Dermatol Ther. 2022;35(9):e15636. https://doi.org/10.1111/dth.15636. Epub 2022 Jul 27.
11. Rinvoq. Package insert. Abbvie; 2019–2022. Updated January 2022.
12. Perche PO, Cook MK, Feldman SR. Abrocitinib: a new FDA-approved drug for moderate-to-severe atopic dermatitis. https://doi-org.ucsf.idm.oclc.org/101177/10600280221096713 [Internet]. 2022 [cited 2022 Dec 23];57(1):86–98. Available from: https://journals-sagepub-com.ucsf.idm.oclc.org/doi/10.1177/10600280221096713?url_ver=Z39.88-2003&rfr_id=ori%3Arid%3Acrossref.org&rfr_dat=cr_pub++0pubmed
13. Ytterberg SR, Bhatt DL, Mikuls TR, Koch GG, Fleischmann R, Rivas JL, Germino R, Menon S, Sun Y, Wang C, Shapiro AB, Kanik KS, Connell CA, ORAL Surveillance Investigators. Cardiovascular and cancer risk with tofacitinib in rheumatoid arthritis. N Engl J Med. 2022;386(4):316–26. https://doi.org/10.1056/NEJMoa2109927.

14. Upadacitinib for rheumatoid arthritis. Aust Prescr 2020;43(5):178–179. doi: https://doi.org/10.18773/austprescr.2020.053. Epub 2020 Aug 6.
15. Nash P, Kerschbaumer A, Dörner T, et al. Points to consider for the treatment of immune-mediated inflammatory diseases with Janus kinase inhibitors: a consensus statement. Ann Rheum Dis. 2021;80:71–87.
16. Tsakok T, Woolf R, Smith CH, Weidinger S, Flohr C. Atopic dermatitis: the skin barrier and beyond. Br J Dermatol. 2019;180(3):464–74.

# Chapter 17
# Treatment of Pediatric AD

Regina-Celeste Ahmad

**Case Title** "A 14-year-old male with widespread, symmetric worsening pruritic rash"

**Case**

A 14-year-old African American male presented for teledermatology consultation during winter season with a worsening progressive pruritic eruption on his neck, arms, and legs for the past year causing considerable sleep disruption. Despite poor video quality, it was apparent the patient had a diffuse symmetric mildly erythematous to violaceous papules and thin plaques on the cheeks, hyperpigmentation of the anterior and posterior neck, and antecubital and popliteal fossae. The mother reported a history of intermittent focal itchy rashes off and on since childhood with worsening during winter season, but never this extensive. The past medical history was significant for untreated allergic rhino-conjunctivitis since childhood with prior positive skin prick testing for multiple indoor and outdoor allergens. There was a family history of seasonal allergies, but no asthma or atopic dermatitis (AD). His skin care routine consisted of fragranced Dove bar soap and Aveeno lotion which he applied daily all over his body including to flared areas. His pediatrician recently prescribed hydrocortisone 1% cream for his face and hydrocortisone 2.5% cream for his body twice daily for 2 weeks only. He experienced no improvement with the hydrocortisone on his face and very mild improvement on the body with rapid flaring once the topical corticosteroids (TCS) were stopped. Upon further questioning, patient had been using TCS to treat his condition off and on for years but had never seen a dermatologist. He had never been prescribed a non-steroidal topical therapy, including topical calcineurin inhibitors (TCIs).

R.-C. Ahmad (✉)
University of California, San Francisco, USA
e-mail: Regina-Celeste.Ahmad@ucsf.edu





N. Brownstone et al. (eds.), *Clinical Cases in Atopic Dermatitis*, Clinical Cases in Dermatology, https://doi.org/10.1007/978-3-031-52147-8_17

While AD was suspected, the sudden worsening raised concern for another etiology including contact dermatitis and secondary infection. The patient was brought into clinic for an in-person visit, and physical examination revealed a skin type V/VI male with much more extensive scaly erythematous thin plaques with numerous overlying dry excoriations than were appreciated during the virtual visit, involving over 40% total body surface area. During confidential assessment, patient reported smoking marijuana regularly, and father smoked cigarettes at home. The patient was asked to stop the fragranced soap, and switch to a non-foaming cleanser along with all hypoallergenic products at home. Smoking cessation counseling was performed, and the negative impact of both first and second-hand smoke on general health as well as worsening of his AD was discussed. He was prescribed fluocinonide ointment (class II topical steroid) for active areas on the body and hydrocortisone 2.5% ointment (class VII) for the face and neck to cycle for 2 weeks and then switch to tacrolimus 0.03% ointment (a TCI). He was also prescribed sedating antihistamines to use sparingly for sleep disturbance. Patient was also referred for patch testing. Patient initially improved on TCS but continued to flare when off TCS. The family was not able to obtain TCI for many weeks due to insurance delays, and then ultimately patient admitted to non-compliance with TCI after it was received. Phototherapy was advised given severity and inability to control condition on topical therapy. However, due to transportation and work constraints, they ultimately declined. Dupilumab injections were initiated, and patient experienced significant improvement in both pruritus and extent of rash within 1–2 months after initiation.

**Board Review Question**

What systemic medication(s) are currently FDA-approved for pediatric atopic dermatitis?

A. Cyclosporine
B. Dupilumab
C. Methotrexate
D. Azathioprine
E. Upadacitinib

## Main Text

Moderate-to-severe pediatric AD can be challenging to recognize and has a significant impact on quality of life for patients and caregivers, with increased likelihood of persistence into adulthood, along with numerous comorbidities [1, 2]. The differential diagnosis of severe pediatric AD includes other chronic dermatoses like allergic and irritant contact dermatitis, psoriasis, immunodeficiencies, genodermatoses, infections, metabolic disease, and rarely cutaneous T-cell lymphoma. The diagnosis of AD is made clinically based on the presence of a chronic, relapsing eczematous dermatitis with associated pruritus [3]. Thorough knowledge of the differences between pediatric and adult AD are essential in making informed diagnostic and therapeutic interventions [4]. Generally, in pediatric AD medical history will be positive for classic age-specific patterns with onset in infancy or childhood. However, when initial presentation is severe or atypical or the diagnosis is in doubt, a skin biopsy and additional workup are appropriate. This is particularly relevant in skin color where papular and nummular subtypes of atopic dermatitis prevail and misdiagnosis may be more likely to occur. Additionally, the full extent of disease activity may be under appreciated in darker skin types without adequate training. Furthermore, while virtual visits may improve access to specialists and provide potentially similar outcomes in the management of chronic skin dermatoses, initial in-person visits are advised in cases of moderate-to-severe AD for the reasons outlined above.

Most pediatric AD can be managed effectively with topical therapy, and TCS remain the mainstay of treatment for majority of AD regardless of age, as well as the most effective "rescue" treatment [5]. TCS may also be applied less frequently as a proactive strategy for disease management in between flares. TCIs are also effective and safe in pediatric AD, though their widespread use in primary care settings continues to be limited, possibly in part due to difficultly explaining black box (BB) warnings and burden of prior authorizations. Safe off-label use in ages less than 2 years is well-supported, and proactive use of TCIs in recurrent areas two to three times weekly is recommended to prevent relapse [5, 6]. While crisaborole (Eucrisa), a topical PDE4 inhibitor, is a promising alternative non-steroidal medication approved down to age 3 months, its mainstream use is still limited by cost and application site discomfort for many pediatric patients [7, 8]. The first topical Janus kinase (JAK) inhibitor ruxolitinib (Opzelura) cream was approved in 2022 for pediatric and adult AD ages 12 and older. Topical JAK inhibitors have demonstrated efficacy and safety in multiple longer-term studies for pediatric and adult AD [9]. Unfortunately, widespread use of ruxolitinib cream is also currently limited by its prohibitive cost and lack of insurance coverage, which disproportionately impacts minority and skin of color groups typically suffering from more severe AD.

AD has historically been undertreated by primary care providers (PCPs) who are generally the first medical professionals to see AD patients. In a review of PCP management practices across all AD severities, there was a lack of adherence to national guidelines including a tendency to prescribe mainly low potency TCS, very limited use of TCIs, over-prescribing of antibiotics, and ongoing use of non-sedating antihistamines which are known to be ineffective in managing AD-associated pruritus [10]. Current guidelines advise against topical anti-staphylococcal treatments aside from dilute bleach baths and intranasal mupirocin in appropriate patients [5]. Judicious use of oral antibiotics is advised only for overt clinical signs of bacterial infection, not simply colonization [11]. Intermittent use of bedtime oral sedating antihistamines may be beneficial in managing sleep disturbance associated with moderate-to-severe AD, though adequate skin-directed care is still paramount. Non-sedating antihistamines are not advised for routine use in AD in the absence of environmental allergies or urticaria. Additionally, there is no evidence to support the use of topical antihistamines in AD. In the case of moderate-to-severe disease, prompt referral to a specialist familiar with managing pediatric AD is critical.

The decision to initiate systemic therapy for moderate-to-severe pediatric AD requires a personalized patient-centered approach that includes the preferences of patient/caregiver, impact on quality of life, workup for alternative diagnoses and co-infection, evaluation for and avoidance of triggers, a trial of phototherapy if appropriate, and appropriate training of patient/caregivers [12]. Prior to initiation of systemic treatment, all patients should have undergone an adequate trial of multimodal topical therapy and regular moisturizing. This includes the use of TCS as well as topical non-steroidal options along with gentle skin care. Wet wrap therapy with TCS and even hospitalization are appropriate to consider during acute severe flares. Additional factors to consider in the workup of severe or recalcitrant pediatric AD include assessment of airborne triggers such as environmental allergens, smoke, or air pollution, as well as medication non-compliance and patient/caregiver burnout.

In addition to adequate skin-directed care and elimination of potential contact irritants, patch testing for contact allergens should be strongly considered in all cases of moderate-to-severe pediatric AD. Pediatric contact dermatitis is more common than previously thought, likely in part due to increased sensitization and limited testing previously available or performed on children. Patch testing is safe for children and can be a useful tool in ruling out other etiologies particularly in the setting of recalcitrant or worsening dermatitis, a new distribution, flaring after cessation of topical therapy, or severe disease [13]. Notably, some common pediatric contact allergens are not part of the standard pediatric testing trays. With appropriate gentle skin care and elimination of potential contact irritants/allergens, a subset of severe cases may improve sufficiently without the need for systemic treatment.

Phototherapy, specifically narrow-band UVB, is considered both safe and effective and has been generally recommended as second-line treatment after topical therapy for moderate-to-severe AD [11]. However, widespread use in the pediatric population is impractical due to lack of sufficient access to centers trained to treat pediatric patients, limited cooperativity in younger ages, and the double burden of frequently missed school and work secondary to bi- or tri-weekly treatments [14]. Severe pediatric AD has been historically undertreated given the only systemic medications available until recently are used off-label in pediatric patients and are associated with risk of severe adverse events. While systemic corticosteroids have been commonly used to treat severe AD flares, this approach is not advised given risk of rebound and high-risk side effects [11]. Cyclosporine, methotrexate, mycophenolate mofetil, and azathioprine have all been used for moderate-to-severe pediatric AD with efficacy, though limited comparative data exists [15]. The frequent laboratory monitoring required for these agents due to risks of significant toxicity is an additional barrier to treatment in pediatric patients. Guidelines have previously been published on the use of phototherapy and these off-label systemic therapies in pediatric and adult AD [11].

The past 6 years have been a boon for options in the management of moderate-to-severe pediatric and adult AD, beginning with dupilumab (Dupixent), a humanized monoclonal antibody inhibiting IL-4 and IL-13 cytokine signaling, as the first FDA-approved biologic medication for adult AD in 2017. It has been recommended by experts as the first-line systemic agent for moderate-to-severe AD in adults [16]. Common side effects include injection site reactions, herpes infections, and conjunctivitis, though increasing reports of hypereosinophilia and facial dermatitis have been appreciated in post-trial reports. Dupilumab initially received pediatric approval for ages 12 and older in 2019 and down to age 6 months as of 2022. A recent systematic review of randomized control trials for dupilumab found that most patients achieved greater than 75% clearance of disease and significant improvements in itch with adverse effects similar to placebo within 16 weeks, though controlled data remains fairly limited in the pediatric population [17, 18]. Real-world data suggests dupilumab has continued to demonstrate efficacy and a favorable safety profile in the pediatric population [18, 19]. Pediatric dosing for dupilumab is weight based, and injections are given between every 2 and 4 weeks. While no routine laboratory monitoring is needed, barriers to this therapy in the pediatric population include need for frequent injections and insurance step therapy requirements. A new biologic, tralokinumab (Adbry), was approved for use in adults in 2021 and works by blocking the IL-13 receptor. In two trials, tralokinumab demonstrated 75% improvement in 25.0% and 33.2% of patients by 16 weeks vs 12.7% and 11.4% on placebo [20]. Common side effects reported were mild and similar to dupilumab, including injection site reactions, upper respiratory infections, conjunctivitis, and eosinophilia. Other biologics and small molecule inhibitors targeting TH2 cytokine signaling as well as pro-inflammatory and itch pathways are in the pipeline for AD.

Oral JAK inhibitors, previously used mainly in rheumatologic conditions, have seen a recent revolution in their application to dermatologic diseases including AD. Two oral JAK inhibitors (upadacitinib and abrocitinib) were approved for moderate-to-severe adult AD in 2022, and upadacitinib was also simultaneously approved for moderate-to-severe pediatric AD in ages 12 and older [21–23]. Two separate trials evaluated response to upadacitinib in adolescents and found that with 15 mg daily dosing 38% and 42% achieved skin clearance at 16 weeks, with a similar percentage experiencing significant improvement in itch [21, 22]. Additionally, 71% and 67% achieved at least 75% skin clearance at 16 weeks. Pediatric trials for other oral JAK inhibitors are underway, though comparative data of different oral JAK inhibitors are not yet available. A comparative trial of dupilumab with abrocitinib in adults suggests more rapid onset of action with the latter in terms of both skin clearance and pruritus measures, though it is unclear if there is superiority overall [24]. A significant practical advantage of JAK inhibitors over dupilumab is the oral route of administration as injection medications are particularly challenging to give in the pediatric population. Despite these promising results, oral JAK inhibitors have significant safety concerns garnering them a BB warning, namely, increased risk of serious infections, malignancy, severe cardiovascular events, and mortality. These side effects are most prevalent in older adults with cardiovascular comorbidity. Regardless, the BB warning and ongoing safety concerns will most likely delay their acceptance for pediatric AD by physicians and families. Additional barriers to use of oral JAK inhibitors in the pediatric population include need for frequent laboratory monitoring and insurance coverage concerns.

While these recently approved systemic treatments are a huge step in improving our management of moderate-to-severe pediatric AD, ongoing use of concomitant topical therapy was shown in all trials to improve outcomes. Many questions remain regarding use of these new systemic agents for pediatric AD, including the need for comparative trials and sub-analyses on which subsets of AD patients may benefit from one agent over another. Additionally, it is unclear if or when these medications can be stopped once initiated, why the effect wanes over time for some patients, and what the long-term effects are when initiated in the pediatric population. With advances in precision medicine for AD, there is hope these questions may be answered, though for many patients the primary barrier to adequate care in severe pediatric AD remains access to specialists and insurance coverage of newer therapeutics.

Finally, in addition to optimal topical and systemic management for moderate-to-severe pediatric AD, awareness of the significant risk of comorbid diseases is important. A multi-disciplinary approach is particularly beneficial to these patients, given high rates of asthma, allergic rhinoconjunctivitis, food allergies, sleep disturbance, and depression along with other neuropsychiatric conditions [2, 25]. Therapy for severe AD needs to be individualized, and a holistic approach with knowledge of complementary and alternative practices with evidence-based efficacy in AD may strengthen the therapeutic relationship and improve outcomes for this vulnerable population.

Severe pediatric AD, while impacting a minority of pediatric AD patients, has significant and long-lasting impacts on health, ranking among the worst dermatologic conditions with respect to quality of life [1, 2, 26]. Effective management of this chronic condition beginning in infancy and early childhood has far-reaching implications for this vulnerable population not only with respect to decreasing comorbidities but also in potentially preventing progression toward the development of additional atopic disease [4, 27]. The armamentarium for treatment of moderate-to-severe pediatric AD is changing rapidly, and recently approved systemic therapies provide new hope for these patients (Table 17.1) [26]. Given the complexity of this chronic condition, along with its many associated comorbidities, co-management with a dermatologist possessing a thorough knowledge of current guidelines and advanced therapies is essential.

**Table 17.1** Current FDA-approved non-steroidal topical and systemic treatments for pediatric atopic dermatitis as of February 2023

| Medication | FDA indication | Pediatric dosing |
|---|---|---|
| Tacrolimus (Protopic) 0.03% ointment | Ages 2 and older (2000) | Twice daily |
| Tacrolimus (Protopic) 0.1% ointment | Ages 16 and older (2000) | Twice daily |
| Pimecrolimus (Elidel) 1% cream | Ages 2 and older (2001) | Twice daily |
| Crisaborole (Eucrisa) ointment | Ages 3 months and older (2020) | Twice daily |
| Ruxolitinib (Opzelura) 1.5% cream | Ages 12 years and older (2022) | Twice daily |
| Dupilumab (Dupixent) | Ages 6 months and older (2022) | Weight-based ages 5–17<br>• 60 kg or more: 600 mg loading dose and 300 mg every other week<br>• 30 kg to less than 60 kg: 400 mg loading dose and 200 mg every other week<br>• Less than 30 kg: 600 mg loading dose and 300 mg every 4 weeks<br>Weight-based ages 6 months to 5 years: No loading dose<br>• 15–30 kg: 300 mg every 4 weeks<br>• 5–15 kg: 200 mg every 4 weeks |
| Upadacitinib (Rinvoq) | Ages 12 years and older (2022) and at least 40 kg | 15 mg daily |

## Board Review Question Explanation

What systemic medication(s) are currently FDA-approved for pediatric atopic dermatitis?

A. Cyclosporine
B. Dupilumab (correct)
C. Methotrexate
D. Azathioprine
E. Upadacitinib (correct)

## Explanation

Dupilumab was the first FDA approved for moderate-to-severe pediatric AD in 2019 (ages 12 and older) and most recently approved down to age 6 months in 2022. Upadacitinib was FDA-approved for moderate-to-severe pediatric AD in 2022 for ages 12 and older.

**Key Takeaway Points**

- Moderate-to-severe pediatric AD may be underrecognized and is commonly undertreated; a multi-disciplinary approach is required for optimal care.
- The prognosis of pediatric AD may be variable, and initial improvement in childhood does not always negate the potential for severe disease in adolescence or adulthood.
- It is appropriate to consider dupilumab as a first-line systemic agent in pediatric patients if phototherapy is not feasible.
- Oral JAK inhibitors represent a newly available systemic treatment for pediatric AD, though additional prospective long-term data is needed to further establish safety in this population.
- Moderate-to-severe pediatric AD benefits from the expertise of a dermatologist experienced with managing pediatric patients, systemic therapy, and workup for associated comorbidities.

## References

1. Yang EJ, Beck KM, Sekhon S, Bhutani T, Koo J. The impact of pediatric atopic dermatitis on families: a review. Pediatr Dermatol. 2019;36(1):66–71. https://doi.org/10.1111/pde.13727. Epub 2018 Dec 16.
2. Davis DMR, Drucker AM, Alikhan A, Bercovitch L, Cohen DE, Darr JM, Eichenfield LF, Frazer-Green L, Paller AS, Silverberg JI, Singh AM, Sidbury R. American Academy of Dermatology guidelines: awareness of comorbidities associated with atopic dermatitis in adults. J Am Acad Dermatol. 2022;86(6):1335–1336.e18. https://doi.org/10.1016/j.jaad.2022.01.009. Epub 2022 Jan 24.
3. Eichenfield LF, Tom WL, Chamlin SL, Feldman SR, Hanifin JM, Simpson EL, Berger TG, Bergman JN, Cohen DE, Cooper KD, Cordoro KM, Davis DM, Krol A, Margolis DJ, Paller AS, Schwarzenberger K, Silverman RA, Williams HC, Elmets CA, Block J, Harrod CG, Smith Begolka W, Sidbury R. Guidelines of care for the management of atopic dermatitis: section 1. Diagnosis and assessment of atopic dermatitis. J Am Acad Dermatol. 2014;70(2):338–51. https://doi.org/10.1016/j.jaad.2013.10.010. Epub 2013 Nov 27.
4. Ramírez-Marín HA, Silverberg JI. Differences between pediatric and adult atopic dermatitis. Pediatr Dermatol. 2022;39(3):345–53. https://doi.org/10.1111/pde.14971. Epub 2022 Mar 16.
5. Eichenfield LF, Tom WL, Berger TG, Krol A, Paller AS, Schwarzenberger K, Bergman JN, Chamlin SL, Cohen DE, Cooper KD, Cordoro KM, Davis DM, Feldman SR, Hanifin JM, Margolis DJ, Silverman RA, Simpson EL, Williams HC, Elmets CA, Block J, Harrod CG, Smith Begolka W, Sidbury R. Guidelines of care for the management of atopic dermatitis: section 2. Management and treatment of atopic dermatitis with topical therapies. J Am Acad Dermatol. 2014;71(1):116–32. https://doi.org/10.1016/j.jaad.2014.03.023. Epub 2014 May 9.
6. Devasenapathy N, Chu A, Wong M, Srivastava A, Ceccacci R, Lin C, MacDonald M, Wen A, Steen J, Levine M, Pyne L, Schneider L, Chu DK. AAAAI/ACAAI joint task force on practice parameters for atopic dermatitis guideline development group. Cancer risk with topical calcineurin inhibitors, pimecrolimus and tacrolimus, for atopic dermatitis: a systematic review and meta-analysis. Lancet Child Adolesc Health. 2023;7(1):13–25. https://doi.org/10.1016/S2352-4642(22)00283-8. Epub 2022 Nov 10.
7. Luger TA, Hebert AA, Zaenglein AL, Silverberg JI, Tan H, Ports WC, Zielinski MA. Subgroup analysis of crisaborole for mild-to-moderate atopic dermatitis in children aged 2 to < 18 years.

Paediatr Drugs. 2022;24(2):175–83. https://doi.org/10.1007/s40272-021-00490-y. Epub 2022 Mar 16.
8. Martín-Santiago A, Puig S, Arumi D, Rebollo Laserna FJ. Safety profile and tolerability of topical phosphodiesterase 4 inhibitors for the treatment of atopic dermatitis: a systematic review and meta-analysis. Curr Ther Res Clin Exp. 2022;96:100679. https://doi.org/10.1016/j.curtheres.2022.100679. eCollection 2022.
9. Sadeghi S, Mohandesi NA. Efficacy and safety of topical JAK inhibitors in the treatment of atopic dermatitis in paediatrics and adults: a systematic review. Exp Dermatol. 2023;32:599. https://doi.org/10.1111/exd.14753Online ahead of print.
10. Young TK, Glick AF, Yin HS, Kolla AM, Velazquez JJ, Nicholson J, Oza VS. Management of pediatric atopic dermatitis by primary care providers: a systematic review. Acad Pediatr. 2021;21(8):1318–27. https://doi.org/10.1016/j.acap.2021.07.008. Epub 2021 Jul 17.
11. Sidbury R, Davis DM, Cohen DE, Cordoro KM, Berger TG, Bergman JN, Chamlin SL, Cooper KD, Feldman SR, Hanifin JM, Krol A, Margolis DJ, Paller AS, Schwarzenberger K, Silverman RA, Simpson EL, Tom WL, Williams HC, Elmets CA, Block J, Harrod CG, Begolka WS, Eichenfield LF. Guidelines of care for the management of atopic dermatitis: section 3. Management and treatment with phototherapy and systemic agents. American Academy of Dermatology. J Am Acad Dermatol. 2014;71(2):327–49. https://doi.org/10.1016/j.jaad.2014.03.030. Epub 2014 May 9.
12. Simpson EL, Bruin-Weller M, Flohr C, Ardern-Jones MR, Barbarot S, Deleuran M, Bieber T, Vestergaard C, Brown SJ, Cork MJ, Drucker AM, Eichenfield LF, Foelster-Holst R, Guttman-Yassky E, Nosbaum A, Reynolds NJ, Silverberg JI, Schmitt J, Seyger MMB, Spuls PI, Stalder JF, Su JC, Takaoka R, Traidl-Hoffmann C, Thyssen JP, van der Schaft J, Wollenberg A, Irvine AD, Paller AS. When does atopic dermatitis warrant systemic therapy? Recommendations from an expert panel of the International Eczema Council. J Am Acad Dermatol. 2017;77(4):623–33. https://doi.org/10.1016/j.jaad.2017.06.042. Epub 2017 Aug 10.
13. Borok J, Matiz C, Goldenberg A, Jacob SE. Contact dermatitis in atopic dermatitis children-past, present, and future. Clin Rev Allergy Immunol. 2019;56(1):86–98. https://doi.org/10.1007/s12016-018-8711-2.
14. Musters AH, Mashayekhi S, Harvey J, Axon E, Lax SJ, Flohr C, Drucker AM, Gerbens L, Ferguson J, Ibbotson S, Dawe RS, Garritsen F, Brouwer M, Limpens J, Prescott LE, Boyle RJ, Spuls PI. Phototherapy for atopic eczema. Cochrane Database Syst Rev. 2021;10(10):CD013870. https://doi.org/10.1002/14651858.CD013870.pub2.
15. Slater NA, Morrell DS. Systemic therapy of childhood atopic dermatitis. Clin Dermatol. 2015;33(3):289–99. https://doi.org/10.1016/j.clindermatol.2014.12.005. Epub 2014 Dec 8.
16. Boguniewicz M, Alexis AF, Beck LA, Block J, Eichenfield LF, Fonacier L, Guttman-Yassky E, Paller AS, Pariser D, Silverberg JI, Lebwohl M. Expert perspectives on management of moderate-to-severe atopic dermatitis: a multidisciplinary consensus addressing current and emerging therapies. J Allergy Clin Immunol Pract. 2017;5(6):1519–31. https://doi.org/10.1016/j.jaip.2017.08.005. Epub 2017 Sep 29.
17. Koskeridis F, Evangelou E, Ntzani EE, Kostikas K, Tsabouri S. Treatment with dupilumab in patients with atopic dermatitis: systematic review and meta-analysis. J Cutan Med Surg. 2022;26(6):613–21. https://doi.org/10.1177/12034754221130969. Epub 2022 Oct 9.
18. Plachouri KM, Georgiou S. Dupilumab in pediatric dermatology. J Dermatolog Treat. 2022;33(2):682–4. https://doi.org/10.1080/09546634.2020.1789049. Epub 2020 Jul 7.
19. Pagan AD, David E, Ungar B, Ghalili S, He H, Guttman-Yassky E. Dupilumab improves clinical scores in children and adolescents with moderate to severe atopic dermatitis: a real-world, single-center study. J Allergy Clin Immunol Pract. 2022;10(9):2378–85. https://doi.org/10.1016/j.jaip.2022.06.014. Epub 2022 Jun 24.
20. Silverberg JI, Toth D, Bieber T, et al. Tralokinumab plus topical corticosteroids for the treatment of moderate-to-severe atopic dermatitis: results from the double-blind, randomized, multicentre, placebo-controlled phase III ECZTRA 3 trial. Br J Dermatol. 2021;184(3):450–63.

21. Guttman-Yassky E, Teixeira HD, Simpson EL, et al. Once-daily upadacitinib versus placebo in adolescents and adults with moderate-to-severe atopic dermatitis (measure up 1 and measure up 2): results from two replicate double-blind, randomised controlled phase 3 trials. Lancet. 2021;397(10290):2151–68.
22. Reich K, Teixeira HD, de Bruin-Weller M, et al. Safety and efficacy of upadacitinib in combination with topical corticosteroids in adolescents and adults with moderate-to-severe atopic dermatitis (AD up): results from a randomised, double-blind, placebo-controlled, phase 3 trial. Lancet. 2021;397(10290):2169–81.
23. Silverberg JI, de Bruin-Weller M, Bieber T, et al. Upadacitinib plus topical corticosteroids in atopic dermatitis: week 52 AD up study results. J Allergy Clin Immunol. 2021:S0091-6749(21)01212-4. https://doi.org/10.1016/j.jaci.2021.07.036.
24. Reich K, Thyssen JP, Blauvelt A, Eyerich K, Soong W, Rice ZP, Hong HC, Katoh N, Valenzuela F, DiBonaventura M, Bratt TA, Zhang F, Clibborn C, Rojo R, Valdez H, Kerkmann U. Efficacy and safety of abrocitinib versus dupilumab in adults with moderate-to-severe atopic dermatitis: a randomised, double-blind, multicentre phase 3 trial. Lancet. 2022;400(10348):273–82. https://doi.org/10.1016/S0140-6736(22)01199-0.
25. Sidbury R, Tom WL, Bergman JN, Cooper KD, Silverman RA, Berger TG, Chamlin SL, Cohen DE, Cordoro KM, Davis DM, Feldman SR, Hanifin JM, Krol A, Margolis DJ, Paller AS, Schwarzenberger K, Simpson EL, Williams HC, Elmets CA, Block J, Harrod CG, Smith Begolka W, Eichenfield LF. Guidelines of care for the management of atopic dermatitis: Section 4. Prevention of disease flares and use of adjunctive therapies and approaches. J Am Acad Dermatol. 2014;71(6):1218–33. https://doi.org/10.1016/j.jaad.2014.08.038. Epub 2014 Sep 26.
26. Lockhart MK, Siegfried EC. Evolving landscape of systemic therapy for pediatric atopic dermatitis. Dermatol Clin. 2022;40(2):137–43. https://doi.org/10.1016/j.det.2021.12.002.
27. Paller AS, Spergel JM, Mina-Osorio P, Irvine AD. The atopic march and atopic multimorbidity: many trajectories, many pathways. J Allergy Clin Immunol. 2019;143(1):46–55. https://doi.org/10.1016/j.jaci.2018.11.006. Epub 2018 Nov 17.

# Chapter 18
# Atopic Dermatitis Spectrum Disorder

**Nicholas Brownstone, Caitlin Lawlor, Gillian Kasper, and John Koo**

**Case Title** A 43-year-old male presents with lichenified plaques and excoriations concentrated on wrist, back of neck, and near the ankles

**Case Presentation**
A 43-year-old male presents to your office complaining of intense pruritus. He has been using Clobetasol 0.05% ointment and other topical steroids on a chronic basis for many years. On physical exam, lichenified plaques with excoriations are seen scattered on various parts of the body but are especially evident on the wrist, back of the neck, and near the ankles. You check the medical record and find that he has chronic and relapsing dermatitis frequently involving the antecubital and popliteal fossa; however, this presentation of dermatitis is not visible at this visit. Moreover, on further questioning, the patient reports a history of both asthma and allergic rhinitis. In addition, he reports having food allergies as a child. How would you diagnose this patient's disease, and how would you treat it?

**Board Review Question**
Which of the following is considered a manifestation of atopic dermatitis?

A. Lichen simplex chronicus
B. Prurigo nodularis
C. Ichthyosis vulgaris

N. Brownstone (✉)
Temple University Hospital, Department of Dermatology, Philadelphia, PA, USA

C. Lawlor · G. Kasper
Lewis Katz School of Medicine, Temple University, Philadelphia, PA, USA
e-mail: tuk12347@temple.edu; gillian.kasper@temple.edu

J. Koo
Department of Dermatology, University of California, San Francisco, USA



N. Brownstone et al. (eds.), *Clinical Cases in Atopic Dermatitis*, Clinical Cases in Dermatology, https://doi.org/10.1007/978-3-031-52147-8_18

D. Hand dermatitis
E. Dennie-Morgan folds
F. All of the above

The concept that certain diseases may manifest as a "spectrum" of disorders has never been introduced to the specialty of dermatology. However, understanding this concept and adapting it where appropriate may significantly improve both diagnostic clarity of dermatologic diseases and therapeutic effectiveness [1]. Atopic dermatitis (AD) is impressive in its heterogenous clinical manifestations [2, 3]. AD not only presents differently according to the patient's age, ethnic background/skin phototype, etc., but it is also associated with many different clinical features which have been considered critical for making the diagnosis of AD (see Table 18.1). These manifestations range from hand dermatitis, ichthyosis vulgaris, and Dennie-Morgan folds to the residual sequelae of chronic itching and scratching, such as prurigo nodularis and lichen simplex chronicus (LSC). With more than 40 different clinical manifestations of atopic dermatitis, it is not surprising that the field of dermatology has created more than ten different diagnostic criteria for AD utilizing different combinations of these various manifestations [4] (Table 18.2).

In the field of psychiatry, this type of ambiguity is avoided by the understanding that some disorders present as a spectrum of disease, while other disorders have a much more limited heterogeneity. For example, in the International Classification of Diseases (ICD)-10, there is an officially recognized diagnosis of "autism spectrum disorder." There is also a diagnosis of obsessive-compulsive spectrum disorder with the understanding that not all manifestations meet any particular diagnostic criteria noted in the DSM-5. This concept of a spectrum disorder is widely recognized by official nosology; for example, "autism spectrum disorder" cannot be denied reimbursement as stated in ICD-10. This allows the providers help patients get optimal access to care.

The concept that AD as a spectrum disorder has been introduced by the senior author (JK) in collaboration with Daniel Butler, MD several years ago [5]. Following that, a consensus meeting was held involving ten key opinion leaders in atopic

**Table 18.1** Eczematous disorders that may be related to atopic dermatitis

| Primary manifestations |
|---|
| Chronic hand eczema |
| Nummular eczema |
| Eyelid dermatitis |
| Dyshidrotic eczema |
| Nipple eczema |
| Asteatotic eczema |
| Gestational eczema |
| Eczema and pruritus of the elderly |
| **Secondary manifestations** |
| Lichen simplex chronicus |
| Prurigo nodularis |

**Table 18.2** Signs and symptoms of atopic dermatitis (reproduced with permission from Vakharia PP, Chopra R, Silverberg JI. Systematic Review of Diagnostic Criteria Used in Atopic Dermatitis Randomized Controlled Trials. *Am J Clin Dermatol.* 2018;19 (1):15–22. doi:10.1007/s40257-017-0299-4)

| | Diagnostic criteria | | | | | | | | | |
|---|---|---|---|---|---|---|---|---|---|---|
| Signs and symptoms | AAD [7] | DARC [8] | Diepgen [9] | HR [10] | ISAAC [11] | JDA [12] | KT [13] | Millenium [14] | SL [15] | UK [16] |
| Pruritus | x | x | | x | x | x | x | x | x | x |
| Age-related or typical distribution (elbows, knees, wrists, ankles, face, neck, hands, arms, legs, trunk) | x | x | | | x | x | x | x | x | x |
| Chronic or chronically relapsing course | x | x | | x | x | x | x | x | x | |
| Personal or family history of atopy (asthma, atopic dermatitis, allergic rhinitis) | x | | x | x | | | x | | x | x |
| Xerosis | x | | x | x | | | x | | x | x |
| Early age of onset | x | | | x | | | x | | x | x |
| Keratosis pilaris | x | | x | x | | | x | | | |
| Palmar hyperlinearity | x | | x | x | | | x | | | |
| White dermographism or delayed blanching | x | | x | x | | | x | | | |
| Dennie-Morgan infraorbital fold | x | | x | x | | | | | | |
| Elevated serum IgE | | | x | x | | | x | | | |
| Facial pallor/ erythema | x | | | x | | | x | | | |
| Food intolerance | | | x | x | | | x | | | |
| Ichthyosis | x | | | x | | | x | | | |
| Intolerance to wool or lipid solvents | | | x | x | | | | | x | |
| Itch when sweating | | | x | x | | | | | x | |
| Lichenification | x | | | | | x | x | | | |
| Orbital darkening | x | | | x | | | x | | | |
| Perifollicular accentuation | x | | | x | | | x | | | |
| Pityriasis alba | x | | x | x | | | | | | |

(continued)

**Table 18.2** (continued)

| Signs and symptoms | Diagnostic criteria | | | | | | | | | |
|---|---|---|---|---|---|---|---|---|---|---|
| | AAD [7] | DARC [8] | Diepgen [9] | HR [10] | ISAAC [11] | JDA [12] | KT [13] | Millenium [14] | SL [15] | UK [16] |
| Cheilitis | | | x | x | | | | | | |
| Course influenced by environmental or emotional factors | | | | x | | | | | x | |
| Immediate (type I) skin test reactivity | | | | x | | | x | | | |
| Prurigo | x | | | | | x | | | | |
| Recurrent or allergic conjunctivitis | | | | x | | | x | | | |
| Tendency toward cutaneous infections or impaired cell-mediated immunity | | | | x | | | x | | | |
| Tendency toward non-specific hand or foot dermatitis | | | | x | | | x | | | |
| Allergen-specific IgE | | | | | | | | x | | |
| Anterior neck folds | | | | x | | | | | | |
| Anterior subcapsular cataracts | | | | x | | | | | | |
| Auricular rhagades | | | x | | | | | | | |
| Cradle cap | | | x | | | | | | | |
| Crusting | | | | | | x | | | | |
| Dyshidrosis | | | x | | | | | | | |
| Erythema or infiltrated erythema | | | | | | x | | | | |
| Exudation | | | | | | x | | | | |
| Hertoghe sign | | | x | | | | | | | |
| Keratoconus | | | | x | | | | | | |
| Nipple eczema | | | | x | | | | | | |
| Papules or vesiculopapules | | | | | | x | | | | |
| Perleche sign | | | x | | | | | | | |
| Photophobia | | | x | | | | | | | |

**Table 18.2** (continued)

| | Diagnostic criteria | | | | | | | | | |
|---|---|---|---|---|---|---|---|---|---|---|
| Signs and symptoms | AAD [7] | DARC [8] | Diepgen [9] | HR [10] | ISAAC [11] | JDA [12] | KT [13] | Millenium [14] | SL [15] | UK [16] |
| RAST screening inhalant allergy | | | x | | | | | | | |
| Scaling | | | | | | x | | | | |
| Sleeplessness | | | | | x | | | | | |
| Symmetrical distribution | | | | | | x | | | | |

*DARC* Danish Allergy Research Centre, *Diepgen* Dipegen atopy score, *HR* Hanifin and Rajka, *IgE* Immunoglobulin E, *ISAAC* International study of asthma and allergies in childhood, *JDA* Japanese Dermatological Association, *Kang* Kang and Tian, *RAST* Radioallergosorbent test, *SL* Schultz-Larsen, *UK* UK refinement of Hanifin and Rajka criteria

dermatitis and psoriasis with the conclusion that AD is in fact a spectrum disorder. Adapting this terminology of "atopic dermatitis spectrum disorder" may eliminate the confusion that results from the presence of the more than ten different diagnostic criteria published in the medical literature. The degree of agreement among the ten key opinion leaders was extremely high; using a modified Delphi method, with a perfect agreement on every statement giving a score of 9.0, the actual agreement among the ten panelists turned out to be 8.8 [6].

The practical implication of adopting this concept and the terminology of "atopic dermatitis spectrum disorder" is numerous and ultimately benefits the patient. First, the deep understanding that atopic dermatitis has more than 40 different clinical manifestations, any of which can appear in the same patient at different times, may lead to a more accurate diagnosis being made for that patient. Dermatologists frequently need to rush through a busy clinic, and it is not unusual for a dermatologist or other dermatology provider increasingly having to see more patients in less time. This can lead to misdiagnoses in a "knee jerk" manner instead of investigating whether there is an underlying broader diagnosis responsible for the visible manifestation for the particular visit. For example, a patient who has been compliant with topical therapy for AD may one day show up to the clinic with LSC being the only visible manifestation for that visit. If the dermatology provider were to simply put the visit diagnosis as "LSC," because that is all he or she sees, then the fact that this is only one manifestation of underlying chronic atopic dermatitis might be entirely missed.

Just as importantly, all the different FDA-approved therapeutic options for AD, ranging from biologics to JAK inhibitors, erroneously become "off label" and inaccessible due to this reflexive misdiagnosis. As all healthcare providers should know, if a particular clinical presentation is just one element of a broader underlying disorder, the healthcare provider is not supposed to use the diagnosis based on that one element but must use the diagnosis of the underlying broader disease. For example, in psychiatry, if a patient with chronic schizophrenia happens to develop an erroneous idea that he or she is infested with parasites, the proper and accurate diagnosis is not delusions of parasitosis but still schizophrenia (the underlying broader disease responsible for the delusions).

Therefore, when a dermatology provider is confronted with a patient who only shows one of the more than 40 different manifestations of AD, it is critically important for the sake of an accurate diagnosis that the provider spends a few more minutes asking the patient the following questions: (1) Did the patient have other rashes in the past? (2) Does the patient have asthma, allergic rhinitis, food allergies, etc.? (3) Is there any family history of AD or other atopic disorders? If the patient turns out to be an atopic dermatitis patient who happened to show only a limited presentation of AD for this visit based on these questions, it is important to not put that limited manifestation as the visit diagnosis; instead, for better accuracy, atopic dermatitis should be recorded as the visit diagnosis. Moreover, in the notes, it is important to document that the patient has "atopic dermatitis spectrum disorder" presenting with whatever the limited manifestation is observed for that visit, such as LSC. Proceeding the consensus meeting mentioned above, several of the key opinion leaders have documented in this style and anecdotally reported that there has been no push back from the payers most likely because this is the more accurate diagnosis. Most importantly, this approach will not unfairly deny access to all the AD medications we have available for the patients who often present with partial and different manifestations of AD at each visit.

**Board Review Question Explanation**

Which of the following is considered a manifestation of atopic dermatitis?

A. Lichen simplex chronicus
B. Prurigo nodularis
C. Ichthyosis vulgaris
D. Hand dermatitis
E. Dennie-Morgan folds
F. All of the above (correct)

**Explanation**

Atopic dermatitis (AD) is an impressively heterogeneous disease in its clinical manifestations. AD not only presents differently according to the patient's age, ethnic background/skin phototype, etc., but it is also associated with many different clinical features which have been considered critical for making the diagnosis of AD (see Table 18.1).

**Key Takeaway Points**

- The concept that certain diseases in dermatology may manifest as a "spectrum" of disorders has never been introduced to the specialty of dermatology.
- AD not only presents differently according to the patient's age, ethnic background/skin phototype, etc., but it is also associated with many different clinical features which have been considered critical for making the diagnosis of AD.
- The practical implication of adopting this concept and the terminology of "atopic dermatitis spectrum disorder" is numerous and ultimately benefits the patient.
- A consensus meeting was held involving ten key opinion leaders in atopic dermatitis and psoriasis with the conclusion that AD is in fact a spectrum disorder.

## References


1. Nakamura T, Haider S, Colicino S, et al. Different definitions of atopic dermatitis: impact on prevalence estimates and associated risk factors. Br J Dermatol. 2019;181(6):1272–9. https://doi.org/10.1111/bjd.17853.
2. Leung DYM. Atopic dermatitis: age and race do matter! J Allergy Clin Immunol. 2015;136(5):1265–7. https://doi.org/10.1016/j.jaci.2015.09.011.
3. Tavecchio S, Angileri L, Pozzo Giuffrida F, Germiniasi F, Marzano AV, Ferrucci S. Efficacy of dupilumab on different phenotypes of atopic dermatitis: one-year experience of 221 patients. J Clin Med. 2020;9(9):2684. https://doi.org/10.3390/jcm9092684.
4. Vakharia PP, Chopra R, Silverberg JI. Systematic review of diagnostic criteria used in atopic dermatitis randomized controlled trials. Am J Clin Dermatol. 2018;19(1):15–22. https://doi.org/10.1007/s40257-017-0299-4.
5. Butler DC, Koo J. Atopic dermatitis spectrum disorder: new conceptualization for the coming new therapeutic era. J Dermatol Treat. 2018;29(8):743–4. https://doi.org/10.1080/09546634.2018.1527433.
6. Butler DC, Simpson E, Guttman-Yassky E, et al. The atopic dermatitis spectrum disorder. Recognizing the clinical heterogeneity in patients with atopic related skin conditions in order to improve therapeutic decision-making and outcomes: an expert panel consensus statement. J Dermatol Treat. 2022;33(4):2397–9. https://doi.org/10.1080/09546634.2021.1966356.
7. Hanifin JM, Cooper KD, Ho VC, et al. Guidelines of care for atopic dermatitis, developed in accordance with the American Academy of Dermatology (AAD)/American Academy of Dermatology Association "administrative regulations for evidence-based clinical practice guidelines". J Am Acad Dermatol. 2004;50(3):391–404.
8. Johnke H, Vach W, Norberg LA, Bindslev-Jensen C, Host A, Andersen KE. A comparison between criteria for diagnosing atopic eczema in infants. Br J Dermatol. 2005;153(2):352–8.
9. Diepgen TL, Sauerbrei W, Fartasch M. Development and validation of diagnostic scores for atopic dermatitis incorporating criteria of data quality and practical usefulness. J Clin Epidemiol. 1996;49(9):1031–8.
10. Hanifin J, Rajka G. Diagnostic features of atopic eczema. Acta Dermato-Venereol. 1980;92:44–7.
11. Asher MI, Keil U, Anderson HR, et al. International study of asthma and allergies in childhood (ISAAC): rationale and methods. Eur Respir J. 1995;8(3):483–91.
12. Tagami H. Japanese Dermatological Association criteria for the diagnosis of atopic dermatitis. J Dermatol. 2002;29(6):398.
13. Kang KF, Tian RM. Criteria for atopic dermatitis in a Chinese population. Acta Derm Venereol Suppl (Stockh). 1989;144:26–7.
14. Bos JD, Van Leent EJ, Sillevis Smitt JH. The millennium criteria for the diagnosis of atopic dermatitis. Exp Dermatol. 1998;7(4):132–8.
15. Schultz Larsen F, Hanifin JM. Secular change in the occurrence of atopic dermatitis. Acta Derm Venereol Suppl (Stockh). 1992;176:7–12.
16. Williams HC, Burney PG, Hay RJ, et al. The U.K. Working Party's diagnostic criteria for atopic dermatitis. I. Derivation of a minimum set of discriminators for atopic dermatitis. Br J Dermatol. 1994;131(3):383–96.

# Chapter 19
# Infection and AD Flares

**Madeleine Kilimnik, Shanthi Narla, and Elizabeth Jones**

## Abbreviations

| | |
|---|---|
| AD | Atopic dermatitis |
| EC | Eczema coxsackium |
| EH | Eczema herpeticum |
| HIV | Human immunodeficiency virus |
| MRSA | Methicillin-resistant *Staphylococcus aureus* |
| MSSA | Methicillin-sensitive *Staphylococcus aureus* |
| SSTI | Skin and soft tissue infection |

**Case Title** An 8-year-old female with pink umbilicated papules overlying eroded eczematous crusted areas

**Case**

An 8-year-old female with a history of mild-moderate atopic dermatitis (AD) presents to the office with an eczema flare. Currently, her AD is managed with daily topical emollients along with topical corticosteroids for acute flares. The patient's

M. Kilimnik
Sidney Kimmel Medical College, Philadelphia, PA, USA

S. Narla
Department of Dermatology, St. Luke's University Health Network, Easton, PA, USA

E. Jones (✉)
Department of Dermatology, Thomas Jefferson University, Philadelphia, PA, USA
e-mail: elizabeth.jones@jefferson.edu



N. Brownstone et al. (eds.), *Clinical Cases in Atopic Dermatitis*, Clinical Cases in Dermatology, https://doi.org/10.1007/978-3-031-52147-8_19

mother states that the child was doing well, and her AD was under control until recently. She suddenly started developing small pink "bumps" on her right arm and flank. Soon afterward, the child began to have an eczema flare in those areas. The bumps are very itchy, and the patient has been scratching her arm significantly. Clinical examination reveals dome-shaped small umbilicated and excoriated pink papules. Other areas are affected by scaly erythematous patches with an overlying honey-colored crust. You diagnose the small pink bumps as molluscum contagiosum. You also discuss with the patient's mother that the crusted eczematous areas may be secondarily infected with a bacteria called *Staphylococcus aureus*. You treat the molluscum according to your office practices and prescribe mupirocin ointment twice a day to areas affected with yellow crust. You review consistent use of a low to medium potency topical corticosteroid to apply to the eczematous areas twice daily for flares. You instruct the mother to call if the crusted areas do not resolve or if the child develops fevers, chills, or other systemic symptoms, in which case you might consider prescribing an antibiotic.

**Board Review Question**
An 8-year-old female with honey-colored crusted lesions surrounding her mouth presents to the clinic. She has a history of AD treated with topical emollients and as-needed topical corticosteroids. The lesions are limited to locations around her mouth. She does not have any fevers, chills, or other systemic symptoms. Her mother asks what the best course of action is for treatment of the new crusted areasP.

A. Allow the infection to self-resolve
B. Use oral cephalexin for the infection
C. Apply topical corticosteroids
D. Use oral acyclovir for the infection
E. Use topical mupirocin for the infection

## Infections in Atopic Dermatitis

The pathogenesis of AD is characterized by the release of type 2 immune cytokines (e.g., Interleukin (IL)-4 and IL-13) which play an important role in skin barrier dysfunction and suppression of antimicrobial peptides (AMP). This shift in immune status predisposes patients with AD to multiple cutaneous and extracutaneous infections [1]. Cutaneous infections can include impetigo, erysipelas, cellulitis, herpes simplex, herpes zoster, warts, molluscum contagiosum, and eczema herpeticum (EH) [2–5]. Extracutaneous, multiorgan, and systemic infections are rare and can include necrotizing fasciitis, acute sinusitis and pharyngitis, bronchitis, croup, acute epiglottitis, pneumonia, aspergillosis, tuberculosis, meningitis, encephalitis, endocarditis, infectious arthropathies, enterocolitis, *clostridium difficile*, pyelonephritis, urinary tract infections, methicillin-sensitive *Staphylococcus aureus* (MSSA), methicillin-resistant *Staphylococcus aureus* (MRSA), and streptococcal, pseudomonal, mycobacterial, fungal, and viral infections [2, 4, 6–9].

Infection in AD is frequent, with 1 study of 1174 AD patients showing 61.4% of patients were either suspected of having a bacterial infection or very likely had one. AD, compared to other dermatoses in the study, had the highest rate of suspected infection [10]. Bacterial superinfection can be a significant burden on patients with AD as it can compound their existing discomfort, pruritus, and the potential psychological side effects of disease symptoms and visibility [11]. Superinfection can be a significant financial burden on the patient. One study showed over one third of AD patients with increased monthly payments were most likely to have persistent skin infections [12].

## *Cutaneous Staphylococcal Infections*

While approximately 20% of healthy patients have been shown to be colonized by *Staphylococcus aureus* (*S. aureus*), between 30 and 100% of AD patients reportedly can be colonized by *S. aurues* [13]. Analysis of inflamed skin from AD patients has shown decreased amounts of *Streptococcus*, *Corynebacterium*, and *Cutibacterium* and the phylum Proteobacteria during an acute AD flare, with a microbial shift toward *S. aureus* [14]. IL-4 and IL-13 inhibit the production of cutaneous AMPs, predisposing AD skin to *Staphylococcus* infections, and Th2 cells facilitate the binding and colonization of *S. aureus* [13].

The most common manifestation of staphylococcal infection in AD patients is impetigo. When a patient scratches their lesions, specifically a patient with AD who is more likely to be colonized by *S. aureus*, it facilitates the superinfection process at wound sites. Bacterial superinfection of existing lesions by *S. aureus* is termed impetiginization, leading to the clinical condition called impetigo. Impetigo can at times be difficult to distinguish from the oozing/weeping that occurs in acute eczematous lesions. Impetigo generally presents with dry, honey-colored crusted lesions overlying an erythematous base and can be treated with a short course of topical mupirocin ointment [15, 16].

Aside from impetigo, in general staphylococcal infections can present as purulent or non-purulent skin and soft tissue infections (SSTI), such as the cellulitis mentioned earlier. Regarding the treatment of staphylococcal infections, a wound culture for these infections should be performed to determine cause and susceptibilities. For hospitalized critically ill patients, vancomycin should be used for MRSA. For MSSA infections, nafcillin or cefazolin can be used. For non-hospitalized patients with a non-purulent infection, an oral beta-lactam which also covers Group A streptococcal species, such as cephalexin, may be used. If purulence or a history of MRSA is present, oral medications such as clindamycin, doxycycline, trimethoprim-sulfamethoxazole (TMP-SMX), and linezolid can be used [16]. For purulent infections, current IDSA guidelines suggest performing an incision and drainage and using empiric TMP-SMX or doxycycline for moderate

**Table 19.1** Outpatient treatment methods for staphylococcal infections

| Infection type | Antibiotics |
|---|---|
| Impetigo | Topical mupirocin |
| Non-purulent SSTI | Oral cephalexin, dicloxacillin, clindamycin, penicillin VK, TMP-SMX +/− amoxicillin, doxycycline +/− amoxicillin, linezolid |
| Purulent SSTI | Incision and drainage +/− any of the following: Topical mupirocin, TMP-SMX, doxycycline |

infections while only using other oral antibiotic options once the bacterial cause is known (Table 19.1) [17].

## *Eczema Herpeticum*

EH is characterized by a herpes simplex viral infection of a pre-existing cutaneous inflammatory condition and is potentially life-threatening. One of the strongest risk factors for EH is atopic dermatitis, with 10–20% of AD patients developing the complication [18]. EH is characterized by punched-out erosions or vesicles and can present with pain, pruritus, fever, malaise, viremia, keratoconjunctivitis, encephalitis, and even septic shock [19].

For diagnosis of EH, a viral culture and PCR sample should be taken from the base of a fresh vesicle, and a Tzanck smear can be performed. Treatment should not be delayed until the results are available, as this can be a fatal condition if left untreated. The mainstay treatment consists of oral acyclovir for immunocompetent patients. Systemic therapy may need to be employed if the infection is rapidly evolving or if the child affected is less than 1 year of age; if the infection surrounds the eye, an ophthalmology evaluation is critical. Due to the often accompanied secondary infection with *S. aureus*, a bacterial culture should be performed, and a prophylactic antibiotic can be initiated [19, 20].

## *Eczema Coxsackium*

Eczema coxsackium (EC), typically caused by the coxsackie A6 and A16 virus, can present similarly to EH and should be considered in the differential [21]. EC presents as vesiculobullous lesions and most commonly affects children with AD. The lesions are usually not pruritic but can be painful. The lesions can present on the hands, feet, torso, groin, and mouth and often localize to areas affected by eczema, becoming confluent along entire areas of the distal extremities. This presentation, specifically lesions on the hands, feet, and mouth, is similar to hand, foot, and mouth disease. EC has been termed "atypical hand, foot, and mouth disease" for this reason [22, 23].

Lesions of EH tend to be more pruritic and painful compared to those of EC, and oral ulcers are much less common in EH as well. Acute vesicles caused by coxsackie viruses are also more of an oval shape compared to the rounded vesicles found in EH [24]. Though fever can occur in EC, it is much more common in EH. To make a diagnosis of EC, a PCR test from a new vesicle or oropharyngeal swab can be used. If a distinction between EH and EC cannot be made, antiviral treatment such as acyclovir can be initiated, though EC will not respond to this. There are no specific medications for EC, but dehydration should be monitored for, as children often have less intake due to painful oral blisters; intravenous hydration may be necessary in certain situations [25, 26].

## *Molluscum Contagiosum*

Molluscum contagiosum is caused by a poxvirus and presents as clustered umbilicated papules on the skin. In one study of 696 patients with molluscum contagiosum, 37.2% had a history of AD. The patients who did have an AD history were also likely to have more molluscum lesions [27]. Molluscum is often diagnosed clinically and via dermoscopy, but a biopsy can be used for diagnosis when necessary. The treatment for molluscum contagiosum varies, and the clinician should use a shared decision-making strategy that best fits the situation. Molluscum is often self-resolving, though can have a lengthy course, so using no treatment is a possibility. Topical cantharidin, retinoids, salicylic acid, podofilox solution, cryotherapy, and even removal of the lesions via curettage or pulsed dye laser are all possibilities. Molluscum contagiosum is, as its name indicates, highly infectious and can spread to different parts of the body as well as to other people, which needs to be taken into account on a case-by-case basis. Education should involve a discussion of avoidance of picking or scratching the bumps to reduce transmission and spread. If an adult patient presents with diffuse molluscum lesions, standard immunocompetency laboratory studies should be ordered, as this can occur in those with human immunodeficiency virus (HIV) and other immunodeficiencies [5, 28].

## Bleach Baths

Historically, bleach baths are a commonly prescribed addition to treatment regimens in atopic dermatitis. Bleach baths have been proposed as a potential adjunctive treatment in patients with moderate-severe AD [29]. Bleach baths can be performed by filling a tub with warm water (~40 gallons) and adding ½ cup of common bleach solution to the bath water (or ¼ cup in half a tub of water). Any sodium hypochlorite 6% solution can be used (e.g., Clorox liquid bleach). Patients can soak in the chlorinated water for 10 min and rinse with fresh lukewarm water, followed by the immediate application of topical emollients or medications [30].

However, the data regarding the efficacy of bleach baths has been conflicting. Of note, in vitro studies found that at the recommended concentration for bleach baths of 0.005% sodium hypochlorite, no bactericidal effect was demonstrated [31]. Moreover, a concentration of at least 0.03% would be needed to have a bactericidal effect against certain strains of *S. aureus*. However, this concentration is cytotoxic to human cells and is much greater than should be used clinically [31]. A systematic review was performed of ten randomized controlled trials addressing bleach baths for AD that enrolled a total of 307 participants (median of mean age 7.2 years, Eczema Area Severity Index (EASI) baseline mean of means 27.57 [median SD, 10.74]) for a median of 6 weeks (range, 4–10) [32]. The results demonstrated that bleach baths probably reduce AD severity (22% vs. 32% EASI-50 [ratio of means 0.78, 95% credible interval 0.59–0.99]; moderate certainty). Adverse events (e.g., dry skin and irritation), itch, patient-reported disease severity, sleep quality, quality of life, and risk of AD flares did not differ between the groups that received bleach baths vs. those who did not (low to very low certainty). Moreover, in patients with moderate-to-severe AD, bleach baths offer 22% relative improvement of clinician-reported severity, and one in ten will likely improve severity by 50%. However, caution needs to be used when interpreting this data given that almost half of the studies were unpublished data and methodologic quality was poor [32].

Of note, the study also found bleach baths may only slightly reduce skin *S. aureus* colonization (risk ratio, 0.89 [95% CI 1.73–109]; low certainty) [32]. This suggests that the efficacy of bleach baths at reducing AD severity may just be from soaking in the water. A previous systematic review and meta-analysis on the efficacy of bleach baths in reducing the severity of AD found that both bleach baths and water baths alone significantly reduced AD severity. Water baths were found to be just as effective as bleach baths at 4 weeks in pooled analyses, and there were no differences in *S. aureus* density in the patients that received bleach baths vs. water [33].

With this recent data, treatment paradigms have started to shift away from the use of bleach baths. However, in some specialty atopic dermatitis clinics or in severe cases, they may still be employed as part of the overall treatment plan.

## Decolonization

There is evidence which suggests that if patients employ strategies to eradicate *S. aureus* from colonizing their bodies, it can mitigate future AD exacerbations. Using topical emollients and corticosteroids on a regular basis, frequent bathing, and avoidance of scratching the pruritic lesions are crucial in this process [19, 34]. Use of mupirocin ointment intranasally twice daily for 5 days has been shown to decrease nasal colonization by *S. aureus*. In a trial analyzing nasal mupirocin use in pre-surgical settings, of the 4030 enrolled patients, of which 891 had *S. aureus* present in their anterior nares, only 4.0% of those who received mupirocin treatment developed post-surgical infections, compared to 7.7% of those who received placebo (odds ratio for infection, 0.49; 95% confidence interval, 0.25–0.92; $P = 0.02$) [35].

Topical retapamulin, povidone-iodine, chlorhexidine gluconate, and the aforementioned sodium hypochlorite bleach baths have also been used as decolonization methods, though with limited data for their support [34]. Of note, there is resistance that can build to these agents, causing them to be less effective and allowing the host to become recolonized [36]. Between 30% and 60% of patients can become recolonized after a decolonization effort. There is a concept called universal decolonization, where all patients, regardless of positive nare swab, undergo decolonization efforts to decrease nosocomial infections among all patients; this has been performed in the ICU setting [34].

**Board Review Question Explanation**

An 8-year-old female with honey-colored crusted lesions surrounding her mouth presents to the clinic. She has a history of AD treated with topical emollients and as-needed topical corticosteroids. The lesions are limited to locations around her mouth. She does not have any fevers, chills, or other systemic symptoms. Her mother asks what the best course of action is for treatment of the new crusted areasP.

A. Allow the infection to self-resolve
B. Use oral cephalexin for the infection
C. Apply topical corticosteroids
D. Use oral acyclovir for the infection
E. Use topical mupirocin for the infection (correct)

**Explanation**

Topical mupirocin is the first-line treatment for impetigo, a common infection which occurs in patients with AD. The majority of cases of impetigo are caused by *Staphylococcus aureus*.

**Key Takeaway Points**

- Infection in AD is extremely common due to barrier dysfunction of the skin.
- Secondary staphylococcal infections in patients must be treated with oral or systemic antibiotics based on severity.
- Bleach baths can be used as an adjunctive method to reduce AD severity, though data is limited and conflicting.
- Decolonization strategies, such as nasal mupirocin, can be used to decrease risk of staphylococcal infections, though recolonization is common.

## References

1. Kim J, Kim BE, Leung DYM. Pathophysiology of atopic dermatitis: clinical implications. Allergy Asthma Proc. 2019;40(2):84–92.
2. Narla S, Silverberg JI. Association between childhood atopic dermatitis and cutaneous, extra-cutaneous and systemic infections. Br J Dermatol. 2018;178(6):1467–8.

3. Silverberg JI, Silverberg NB. Childhood atopic dermatitis and warts are associated with increased risk of infection: a US population-based study. J Allergy Clin Immunol. 2014;133(4):1041–7.
4. Narla S, Silverberg JI. Association between atopic dermatitis and serious cutaneous, multiorgan and systemic infections in US adults. Ann Allergy Asthma Immunol. 2018;120(1):66–72.e11.
5. Olsen JR, Piguet V, Gallacher J, Francis NA. Molluscum contagiosum and associations with atopic eczema in children: a retrospective longitudinal study in primary care. Br J Gen Pract. 2016;66(642):e53–8.
6. Serrano L, Patel KR, Silverberg JI. Association between atopic dermatitis and extracutaneous bacterial and mycobacterial infections: a systematic review and meta-analysis. J Am Acad Dermatol. 2019;80(4):904–12.
7. Strom MA, Silverberg JI. Association between atopic dermatitis and extracutaneous infections in US adults. Br J Dermatol. 2017;176(2):495–7.
8. Ren Z, Silverberg JI. Association of Atopic Dermatitis with Bacterial, fungal, viral, and sexually transmitted skin infections. Dermatitis. 2020;31(2):157.
9. Silverberg J. Associations between atopic dermatitis and other disorders. F1000Res. 2018;7:303. [version 1; peer review: 3 approved].
10. Wang X, Shi XD, Li LF, Zhou P, Shen YW. Classification and possible bacterial infection in outpatients with eczema and dermatitis in China: a cross-sectional and multicenter study. Medicine (Baltimore). 2017;96(35):e7955.
11. Drucker AM. Atopic dermatitis: burden of illness, quality of life, and associated complications. Allergy Asthma Proc. 2017;38(1):3–8.
12. Chovatiya R, Begolka WS, Thibau IJ, Silverberg JI. Impact and associations of atopic dermatitis out-of-pocket health care expenses in the United States. Dermatitis. 2022;33(6S):S43–51.
13. Kim JE, Kim HS. Microbiome of the skin and gut in atopic dermatitis (AD): understanding the pathophysiology and finding novel management strategies. J Clin Med. 2019;8(4):444.
14. Paller AS, Kong HH, Seed P, et al. The microbiome in patients with atopic dermatitis. J Allergy Clin Immunol. 2019;143(1):26–35.
15. Cole C, Gazewood J. Diagnosis and treatment of impetigo. Am Fam Physician. 2007;75(6):859–64.
16. Liu C, Bayer A, Cosgrove SE, Daum RS, Fridkin SK, Gorwitz RJ, Kaplan SL, Karchmer AW, Levine DP, Murray BE, Rybak J, Talan DA, Chambers HF, Infectious Diseases Society of America. Clinical practice guidelines by the Infectious Diseases Society of America for the treatment of methicillin-resistant Staphylococcus aureus infections in adults and children. Clin Infect Dis. 2011;52(3):e18–55.
17. Stevens DL, Bisno AL, Chambers HF, Dellinger EP, Goldstein EJ, Gorbach SL, Hirschmann JV, Kaplan SL, Montoya JG, Wade JC. Practice guidelines for the diagnosis and management of skin and soft tissue infections: 2014 update by the Infectious Diseases Society of America. Clin Infect Dis. 2014;59(2):147.
18. Hsu DY, Shinkai K, Silverberg JI. Epidemiology of eczema herpeticum in hospitalized U.S. children: analysis of a Nationwide cohort. J Invest Dermatol. 2018;138(2):265–72.
19. Wang V, Boguniewicz J, Boguniewicz M, Ong PY. The infectious complications of atopic dermatitis. Ann Allergy Asthma Immunol. 2021;126(1):3–12.
20. Liaw FY, Huang CF, Hsueh JT, Chiang CP. Eczema herpeticum: a medical emergency. Can Fam Physician. 2012;58(12):1358–61.
21. Ventarola D, Bordone L, Silverberg N. Update on hand-foot-and-mouth disease. Clin Dermatol. 2015;33(3):340–6.
22. Mathes EF, Oza V, Frieden IJ, Cordoro KM, Yagi S, Howard R, Kristal L, Ginocchio CC, Schaffer J, Maguiness S, Bayliss S, Lara-Corrales I, Garcia-Romero MT, Kelly D, Salas M, Oberste MS, Nix WA, Glaser C, Antaya R. "Eczema coxsackium" and unusual cutaneous findings in an enterovirus outbreak. Pediatrics. 2013;132(1):e149–57.

23. Kuntz T, Koushk-Jalali B, Tigges C, Silling S, di Cristanziano V, Wieland U, Oellig F, Kreuter A. Atypische hand-Fuß-Mund-Krankheit [Atypical variant of hand-foot-mouth disease]. Hautarzt. 2019;70(12):964–8.
24. Kimmis BD, Downing C, Tyring S. Hand-foot-and-mouth disease caused by coxsackievirus A6 on the rise. Cutis. 2018;102(5):353–6.
25. Bunya VY, Houser K, Yen MT, Lee NG. Eczema herpeticum. EyeWiki; 2022. https://eyewiki.aao.org/Eczema_Herpeticum#cite_note-:6-9. Accessed 13 Jan 2023
26. Trayer J, Gore C. Severe eczema flare and Coxsackie virus. BMJ Case Reports. 2022;15(2):e247656.
27. Berger EM, Orlow SJ, Patel RR, Schaffer JV. Experience with molluscum contagiosum and associated inflammatory reactions in a pediatric dermatology practice. Arch Dermatol. 2012;148(11):1257.
28. Molluscum contagiosum: diagnosis and treatment. American Academy of Dermatology; n.d. https://www.aad.org/public/diseases/a-z/molluscum-contagiosum-treatment. Accessed 13 Jan 2023
29. Boguniewicz M, Fonacier L, Guttman-Yassky E, Ong PY, Silverberg J, Farrar JR. Atopic dermatitis yardstick: practical recommendations for an evolving therapeutic landscape. Ann Allergy Asthma Immunol. 2018;120(1):10–22.e12.
30. Krakowski AC, Eichenfield LF, Dohil MA. Management of atopic dermatitis in the pediatric population. Pediatrics. 2008;122(4):812–24.
31. Sawada Y, Tong Y, Barangi M, et al. Dilute bleach baths used for treatment of atopic dermatitis are not antimicrobial in vitro. J Allergy Clin Immunol. 2019;143(5):1946–8.
32. Bakaa L, Pernica JM, Couban RJ, et al. Bleach baths for atopic dermatitis: a systematic review and meta-analysis including unpublished data, Bayesian interpretation, and GRADE. Ann Allergy Asthma Immunol. 2022;128(6):660–668.e669.
33. Chopra R, Vakharia PP, Sacotte R, Silverberg JI. Efficacy of bleach baths in reducing severity of atopic dermatitis: a systematic review and meta-analysis. Ann Allergy Asthma Immunol. 2017;119(5):435–40.
34. Sharara SL, Maragakis LL, Cosgrove SE. Decolonization of staphylococcus aureus. Infect Dis Clin N Am. 2021;35(1):107–33.
35. Perl TM, Cullen JJ, Wenzel RP, Zimmerman MB, Pfaller MA, Sheppard D, Twombley J, French PP, Herwaldt LA. Mupirocin and the risk of Staphylococcus Aureus Study Team. Intranasal mupirocin to prevent postoperative Staphylococcus aureus infections. N Engl J Med. 2002;346(24):1871–7.
36. McNeil JC, Hulten KG, Kaplan SL, Mason EO. Decreased susceptibilities to retapamulin, mupirocin, and chlorhexidine among Staphylococcus aureus isolates causing skin and soft tissue infections in otherwise healthy children. Antimicrob Agents Chemother. 2014;58(5):2878–83.

# Chapter 20
# Newer Treatments, Treatment Selection, Pipeline Therapies, and Personalized Medicine in Atopic Dermatitis: Where Are We Now?

**James Q. Del Rosso**

**Case Title** An inquisitive young female computer programmer presents with "atopic eczema" for 30 years and is searching for "better control of my itching and recurring rash." She asks, "Is there anything new coming along that works better or any testing that can help decide what treatments may be best for me?"

**Case**

A 32-year-old Asian female presents with a 30-year history of recurrent widespread and markedly pruritic atopic dermatitis. She was born in the United States and lived in Nevada her entire life. Her brother who is 25 years of age also has "atopic eczema" since childhood, but his case is not as severe. She has used various moisturizer products, prescription topical therapies (including corticosteroids, tacrolimus, and crisaborole), intermittent intramuscular corticosteroid injections, and a course of oral cyclosporine **in** the past. The latter therapy helped for a while but was stopped due to severe gingival hyperplasia and concern about chronic immunosuppression. She has undergone patch testing by an experienced dermatologist 2 years ago which did not identify any allergens believed to correlate with her condition. She is very compliant with her treatments and follow-up recommendations. Her skin care and personal use hygiene products have been unchanged for several years as she diligently searched to find products that do not sting, burn, or cause itching or a rash.

Currently she is using dupilumab 300 mg injections every 2 weeks over the past 8 months which have improved the "skin rash" and itching, but she still experiences intermittent flares once every few months which she cannot relate to any triggering factors. Mometasone ointment is used sparingly and intermittently for areas that are most persistent on her extremities. She does not want to continue repeated "cortisone injections" due to concern about side effects, especially as "they only help for

J. Q. Del Rosso (✉)
Touro University Nevada, Henderson, NV, USA



N. Brownstone et al. (eds.), *Clinical Cases in Atopic Dermatitis*, Clinical Cases in Dermatology, https://doi.org/10.1007/978-3-031-52147-8_20

1 or 2 months." Itching associated with flares is often severe, especially on her extremities and neck, and she has difficulty falling or staying asleep on two to three nights a week. She has seen an ophthalmologist for "mild conjunctivitis" which is well controlled overall with OTC eye lubricants twice daily and intermittent use of loteprednol eye drops. Her only medications are oral contraceptives over the past 5 years and **oral** fexofenadine 180 mg daily when needed for "nasal allergies." She has no history of asthma and no known food allergies. Her dermatologist is considering use of an oral Janus kinase (JAK) inhibitor which she is considering but is concerned about how long she will be on it due to potential side effects. There is no personal or family history of cardiac disease, vascular disease, thromboembolism, malignancy, or tuberculosis. She is very inquisitive about what therapies may be coming along and if there are any testing methods to determine what treatments may be best. She has two young children, none with any skin problems to date.

**Board Review Question**
Which of the following binds to OX40L and prevents its interaction with OX40?

A. Dupilumab.
B. Tralokinumab.
C. Amlitelimab.
D. Secukinumab.
E. Ligelizumab.

## Main Text

This case depicts a common course in life for many patients affected by atopic dermatitis (AD). This disorder which commonly starts early in life in predisposed individuals is typified by exacerbations and relative remissions, with many patients experiencing a low-grade eczematous and/or xerotic dermatitis for several days of the year between more severe flares [1–4]. The pathophysiology of AD is complex involving an individualized interplay of genetics, environmental factors, immune dysregulation, and microbial dysbiosis in each affected individual; triggers are often difficult to identify or avoid, and even when some are noted, flares are often inexplicable regarding their cause [5–8]. In many cases, **AD** persists into adulthood, and **some** cases of late-onset AD have been identified [9]. Over time, affected patients typically utilize a variety of over-the-counter products, topical prescription agents, and intermittent "burst" of systemic corticosteroid therapy, and some are treated with phototherapy or conventional systemic immunosuppressive agents, such as cyclosporin and methotrexate [10, 11].

As AD is a chronic and debilitating disease, long-term management is a very important clinical consideration warranting careful consideration of the potential benefits, risks, and limitations of all available treatment options. Many of the conventional topical and systemic therapies used for AD exhibit limitations related to potential safety risks and/or inadequate disease control, supporting a very strong need for newer therapies [12].

In the last several years, injectable monoclonal antibodies (dupilumab, tralokinumab), both of which suppress augmented Th2 inflammation that is often a predominant pathophysiologic component of AD, have been approved for use in moderate to severe AD refractory to prescription topical therapy. These agents have revolutionized the effective management of AD for many affected individuals [13–16]. These monoclonal antibodies exhibit highly favorable efficacy and safety profiles, are amenable to long-term use to both achieve and maintain effective control of AD, and are essentially devoid of major adverse effects and other limitations associated with the conventional systemic immunosuppressive agents [13, 17–19]. More recently, a topical JAK inhibitor (ruxolitinib) **has been approved for mild to moderate AD refractorty to other prescription topical therapies,** and two oral JAK inhibitors (abrocitinib, upadacitinib) have been approved for use in moderate to severe AD refractory to systemic therapy, including a biologic agent [20–22]. Topical **ruxolitinib** offers a non-steroidal option that exhibits a quick onset of effect in reducing pruritus and effective reduction in eczematous lesions and can be safely used at all affected cutaneous sites [22]. Despite being assigned the "boxed warnings" for specific major adverse events (AEs) attributed to oral JAK inhibitors (JAK-1, JAK-2, or JAK-3 inhibition), there is negligible risk of major AEs with appropriate use of ruxolitinib cream to active AD lesions in up to 20% body surface area based on pharmacokinetic evaluation in animals and humans, including maximum use study data [23]. Other novel nonsteroidal topical therapies are also under development for AD, and their availability is anticipated for the near future.

So where are we with the patient we are caring for as described in the case review above? Due to the extensive amount of body surface area involved, initiation of topical ruxolitinib is not viable as a sole recommendation. Other considerations currently available would be changing to tralokinumab from dupilumab. Although data are limited on switching between dupilumab and tralokinumab in either direction, an open-label case report series noted marked improvement in 12 adult patients with AD who were on previous treatment with dupilumab, 4 of whom developed conjunctivitis on dupilumab that did not recur with tralokinumab treatment [24]. More data are needed on switching between monoclonal antibodies for AD.

The consideration of an oral JAK inhibitor is a very realistic consideration in this case, provided the patient accepts the potential risks and follow-ups with appropriate monitoring recommendations at baseline and periodically thereafter. Pivotal clinical studies with individual agents, a systematic review of systemic therapies for AD, and FDA approval of both agents support the favorable efficacy of both **abrocitinib** and upadacitinib in refractory moderate to severe AD in adolescents and adults [20, 21, 25–27]. Data are available to demonstrate superior overall efficacy including faster onset of itch reduction with both upadacitinib and abrocitinib versus **dupilumab;** an incremental increase in efficacy may be seen with either upadacitinib (30 mg daily) or abrocitinib (200 mg daily) after previous treatment with dupilumab for 6 months, offering the option of changing to JAK inhibitor therapy to achieve greater efficacy that is supported by evidence shown in clinical trials [28–31].

The potential for augmented efficacy by switching from dupilumab to **upadacitinib** or abrocitinib is one important consideration. The other considerations are relative safety and laboratory monitoring. A complete review of safety data with oral JAK inhibitors is beyond the scope of this chapter. Multiple publications are available on JAK inhibitor safety. What is important to keep in mind are differences between the individual agents; the treated populations with regard to age, disease state, comorbidities, and other risk factors; and evaluation of long-term data as new information emerges over time [25, 28, 32–36]. Importantly, a primary emphasis behind boxed warnings (for serious infections, major cardiovascular events, malignancy, and thromboembolism) included in FDA-approved labeling with oral JAK inhibitors approved to treat AD and alopecia areata (AA) incorporated data that evaluated use of a pan-JAK inhibitor (tofacitinib) in patients ≥50 years of age treated for rheumatoid arthritis with other risk factors including concomitant use of immunosuppressives such as methotrexate and corticosteroids [26, 27]. Evaluations of AD and AA patients treated with oral JAK inhibitors that inhibit primarily JAK-1/JAK-2 who are younger in mean age and generally devoid of the comorbidities seen in older patients demonstrate a much lower rate of major AEs, including those depicted in the boxed warnings. [33–38] This is an important consideration when discussing potential risks with oral JAK inhibitor therapy such as with the patient described above. Baseline and follow-up clinical and laboratory monitoring recommendations are important to review and are generally not stringent in younger patients without other concomitant risk factors and comorbidities [25–28, 32–36]. See Table 20.1 which outlines suggested monitoring in patients treated for AD with oral JAK inhibitor therapy (JAK1, JAK2, JAK3 inhibition).

A systematic review and meta-analysis suggested that current evidence does not detect an increased risk of venous thromboembolism associated with AD or with

**Table 20.1** Clinical use of oral JAK (1/2/3) inhibitors in atopic dermatitis clinical and laboratory monitoring recommendations

| |
|---|
| • *Patient Selection*—shared discussion of benefit/risk assessment |
| – Exclude: severe infections, malignancy, pregnancy/lactation, VTE[a], other co-morbidities/disease states |
| – Approach consistent with reasonable management of the disease state |
| • *Careful Dosing/Regimen Selection*—consider patient-related factors |
| • *Pre-Treatment Screening/Risk Evaluations* |
| – H&P, CBC, LFTs[b], Renal function, Lipid levels, CPK testing not recommended for routine testing **(individualized determination; clinician and/or patient preference)** |
| – Hepatitis B testing, hepatitis C testing, TB screening, HIV testing (if high risk) |
| – Assess and update vaccination status/Assess risk factors for VTE |
| • *Follow-up Monitoring* |
| – CBC and LFTs at 1 and 3 months and periodically thereafter; serum lipid levels at 3 months and as clinically indicated thereafter |
| – Annual skin exam/skin cancer detection |
| Note: There may be **specific** monitoring differences noted in individual product package inserts |

Adapted from Nash P, et al. Ann Rheum Dis 2020;1-17. doi:10.1136/annrheumdis-2020-218398; FDA-approved package inserts for abrocitinib and upadacitinib for atopic dermatitis.
[a]*VTE* Venous Thromboembolism
[b]*LFTs* Liver Function Tests

treatment with JAK inhibitors (upadacitinib, abrocitinib, baricitinib) [37]. Another report analyzed data regarding AEs of special interest for methotrexate, cyclosporine, and systemic corticosteroids and calculated the incidence of AEs per 100 patient-years for these drugs, including data regarding baseline incidence of AEs in AD and control patients. Results showed that compared to upadacitinib and abrocitinib, traditional systemic therapies for AD demonstrated equal or higher incidence rates for malignancy (except non-melanoma skin cancer), non-melanoma skin cancer, major adverse cardiac events, and venous thromboembolism, although there were some differences among the populations studied among the different traditional systemic agents. Upadacitinib and abrocitinib also exhibited either comparable or lower incidence of malignancy (excluding non-melanoma skin cancer), major adverse cardiac events, and venous thromboembolism, but higher rates of **non-melanoma** skin cancer, in comparison to baseline rates in AD or control patients [38]. The bottom line is that more data are always welcome regarding specific patient populations and their potential associations with efficacy and safety.

What other systemic therapies are in the pipeline for treatment of AD? The complexity of AD pathophysiology and the multiple "circuits" of dysregulation involved in inducing barrier impairment and/or inflammation allow for multiple potential therapeutic targets. Additional monoclonal antibodies that inhibit the effects of IL-13 include lebrikizumab and eblasakimab, the latter an inhibitor of the IL-13 receptor that is in early stages of development. [39, 40] Lebrikizumab is a humanized monoclonal antibody that exhibits high affinity receptor binding to circulating IL-13 [41]. Available clinical trials through phase 3 demonstrate favorable safety and efficacy for eczematous skin lesions and pruritus in adolescents and adults with moderate-to-severe AD; as with tralokinumab, many patients can effectively reduce injection frequency from every 2 weeks to every 4 weeks once a successful response is achieved within the first few months of treatment [42, 43]. Similar to dupilumab and tralokinumab, this agent does not appear to warrant any definitive baseline or periodic laboratory testing, exhibiting a similar favorable safety profile including with long-term data [42, 43]. Additionally, many patients who achieve an effective response within the first few months of lebrikizumab use are able to sustain both EASI-75 reduction and clinically meaningful reduction in pruritus [44].

Another humanized monoclonal antibody in later stages of development is nemolizumab which is an anti-IL-31 receptor α-chain (IL-31RA) monoclonal antibody agent shown to improve symptoms of AD in phase II and phase III studies [39, 45–48]. This agent exhibits a quick onset of action, exhibiting greater efficacy in reducing pruritus than for eczematous lesions of AD, along with a favorable safety profile [45, 47, 48]. The notable finding of greater efficacy for pruritus is supported by the observation that IL-31 receptors are overexpressed on sensory nerves [47]. An additional placebo-controlled 16-week study of nemolizumab in AD used along with topical agents demonstrated significantly greater reduction of pruritus in the actively treated group [46]. More data are needed to determine where this agent will fit in the AD treatment armamentarium.

Several other systemic agents have been evaluated targeting **a variety of** different cytokines, receptors, and other mechanisms, including anti-IgE, anti-IL 5, anti-IL 22, anti-IL 12/23, anti-IL-17, anti-CD20, anti-H4 receptor (anti-H4R), inhibition of immune checkpoint co-stimulatory molecules (anti-OX40; anti-OX40 ligand), PDE4 inhibition, dihomo-gamma-linolenic acid (DGLA), JAK-SYK signaling inhibition, and TSLP binding inhibition [40, 46, 48–54]. Many are supported by limited

**Table 20.2** Selected potential systemic therapies for atopic dermatitis

| Mode of action | Specific agent | Route | Observations |
|---|---|---|---|
| Anti-IL 5 | Mepolizumab | SC | IL-5 is a Th2 cytokine that functions as an eosinophil chemoattractant; mepolizumab is a fully humanized mAb FDA-approved for severe eosinophilic asthma and eosinophilic granulomatosis and polyangiitis; a RCT in AD did not show clinical success or reduction in TARC serum levels compared to placebo, but significant reduction in peripheral blood eosinophil counts was noted in the actively treated group |
| Anti-IgE | Omalizumab | SC | Omalizumab is a recombinant anti-IgE mAb FDA-approved for treatment of asthma and chronic idiopathic urticaria; variable results reported in AD; systematic review and meta-analysis reported <50% of treated patients demonstrated significant clinical outcomes or reduction in pruritus based on several study parameters (EASI, SCORAD, IGA, 2-point NRS reduction); phase 4 study in severe AD in children markedly reduced disease severity and topical corticosteroid use; potential for use in specific subsets with AD |
| | Ligelizumab | SC | Ligelizumab is an anti-IgE mAb with greater binding affinity for IgE; also inhibits binding of IgE to mast cells and basophils; superior to omalizumab in IgE suppression; phase 2 study in AD completed with results unpublished |
| TSLP receptor binding inhibition | Tezepelumab | SC | TSLP is a cytokine produced by keratinocytes/epithelial cells and other cell types; induces Th2 immune response; overexpressed in keratinocytes in acute and chronic AD lesions and high serum levels in children with AD; tezepelumab is a fully human mAb binding TSLP; phase 2a study did not show statistically significant improvements vs placebo is multiple study endpoints (primary and secondary) |
| Anti-IL 22 | Fezakinumab | IV | IL-22 produced by Th22 cells induces epidermal hyperplasia and barrier impairment and promotes T-cell migration into the skin in acute and chronic AD; fezakinumab is a fully humanized anti-IL 22 mAb which modulates keratinocyte proliferation and promotes upregulation of antimicrobial peptides; a phase 2a RCT showed significantly greater response based on multiple efficacy parameters (e.g., IGA SCORAD, BSA) in severe AD as compared to moderate AD; a study assessing baseline IL-22 levels in AD showed that subjects with high levels were responders and those with low levels responded poorly to fezakinumab use; baseline IL-22 levels and disease severity may have potential as predictors of clinical response in AD |

**Table 20.2** (continued)

| Mode of action | Specific agent | Route | Observations |
|---|---|---|---|
| PDE4 inhibition | Apremilast | Oral | PDE4 an intracellular physiologic regulator of inflammation via control of cAMP levels; overexpressed in AD decreases cAMP which enhances inflammation in AD; limited data on efficacy for AD; 40 mg BID with some improvements in EASI scores and biomarker response with improvements not noted with 30 mg BID; side effects a major factor limiting clinical use |
| OX40 ligand (OX40L) inhibition | Amlitelimab | **IV, SC** | Amlitelimab is a human non-depleting mAb that binds to OX40L preventing interactions with OX40; blocks APC (T cell) activation and inhibits OX40L back signaling aiming to restore immune homeostasis (pro- and anti-inflammatory T cell balance); RCTs in AD showed efficacy and reduction in pruritus with efficacy results maintained for 6 months after treatment; sustained reduction in IL-22 noted; available data supports blockade of both Th2 and Th1/17/T22 inflammation; highly favorable safety profile to date |
| OX-40 inhibition | Rocatinlimab | IV, SC | Rocatinlimab is a fully human anti-OX40 mAb under evaluation for AD; inhibition of Th2 inflammation via **marked** depletion of OX40+ activated T cells and diminished clonal T cells; quantitative PCR analysis showed decreased OX40 mRNA expression and downregulation of Th2, Th1/Th17, and Th22-related genes post-treatment; phase 2b RCT showed efficacy with multiple doses with durability of response; post hoc evaluation in head and neck AD noted persistence of therapeutic effect for 5 months post-treatment supported by skin transcriptome analysis; highly favorable safety profile to date |
| Anti-IL 12/23 | Ustekinumab | SC | Ustekinumab is a human mAb that regulates Th1 and Th17/Th22 responses by inhibiting activity of IL-12 and IL-23 via targeting of the shared p40 subunit; FDA-approved in patients ≥6 years of age with plaque psoriasis and in active psoriatic arthritis and in adults with Crohn's disease or ulcerative colitis; in RCTs in adults with AD greater efficacy was noted in subjects on ustekinumab, but the results were not statistically significant |
| Anti-IL 17 | Secukinumab | SC | Secukinumab is a human mAb antagonist of IL-17A; FDA-approved for plaque psoriasis (≥6 years of age), active psoriatic arthritis (>2 years of age), adults with active ankylosing spondylitis **or** non-radiographic axial spondyloarthritis with inflammation, and active enthesitis-related arthritis (≥4 years of age); limited data in AD with a phase 2 trial showing no significant improvement (EASI scores, IGA) |

(continued)

**Table 20.2** (continued)

| Mode of action | Specific agent | Route | Observations |
|---|---|---|---|
| JAK-SYK signaling inhibition | Gusacitinib | Oral | Gusacitinib is a dual inhibitor of JAK and SYK kinases; a phase 1b RCT in AD showed a dose-related response with 40 mg daily and 80 mg daily significantly superior to 20 mg and placebo **in** specific efficacy parameters; more data are needed |
| Dihomo-gamma-linolenic acid (DGLA) | DS-107 | Oral, topical | In a phase 2a RCT superiority of oral DGLA noted over placebo in IGA and pruritus (NRS) for moderate-to-severe AD; in a phase 2b RCT topical DGLA cream 5% showed **statistical** superiority (IGA, EASI-75) over DGLA cream 1% and vehicle for mild-to-moderate AD; more data are needed |

*Abbreviations: AD* Atopic dermatitis, *APC* Antigen-presenting cell, *EASI* Eczema area severity index, *FDA* Food and Drug Administration, *IL* Interleukin, *IV* Intravenous, *mAb* Monoclonal antibody, *NRS* Numerical rating scale (pruritus), *RCT* Randomized controlled trial, *SCORAD* Scoring atopic dermatitis, *TARC* Thymus and activation-regulated chemokine, *TSLP* Thymic stromal lymphopoietin, *SC* Subcutaneous

data to date; however, further studies are likely to be forthcoming with some of these potential therapies for AD [39, 40, 46, 48–54]. Table 20.2 outlines many of these other systemic agents that have undergone evaluation for AD. An important observation is that many agents with different primary modes of action have exhibited efficacy for AD in some early trials, although some have failed to meet primary endpoints, have demonstrated conflicting results among different studies, or appear to be of therapeutic benefit in specific sub-populations of study subjects. Studies with biologic agents that inhibit IL-17 (e.g., secukinumab) or IL-12/23 (e.g., ustekinumab) support that inhibition of these cytokines appears to play a much greater role for treatment of psoriasis than for AD, although specific subsets of AD may respond favorably to their use [55]. These variable outcomes support the heterogenous and complex nature of AD pathophysiology and the need for further research to accurately differentiate specific AD phenotypes and endotypes which will likely lead to a more personalized and accurate approach to treatment selection.

Recognition of the important role of co-stimulatory molecules (immune checkpoint molecules), specifically the OX40-OX40L axis, in T helper effector cell differentiation is another promising target pathway for therapeutic intervention [49–52]. OX40 is expressed on T cells, and OX40 ligand (OX40L) is expressed on antigen-presenting cells (e.g., dendritic cells); ligation of OX40 by OX40L produces the sustained activation and expansion of effector T and effector memory T cells (without activity in naïve and resting memory cells) which appears to be vital in promoting Th2 immune deviation common to AD [49, 51]. Several cytokines including TSLP, IL-25, and IL-33 stimulate specific immune cells to express OX40L and upregulate Th2 differentiation [49]. The OX40-OX40L axis is a major focus of research on the pathophysiology of AD and development of therapeutic agents that target these co-stimulatory molecules, such as amlitelimab (anti-OX40L) and rocatinlimab (anti-OX40) [49–52].

A major goal in our understanding of the pathophysiology and optimal management of AD is for researchers to sort through the vast array of cytokines, chemokines, and other "messengers" and to ultimately differentiate which are truly operative, which may serve as predictive biomarkers of disease activity and/or treatment response and which are only innocent bystanders that play little or no role in AD. The complexity of this challenge is that different phenotypes of AD may exhibit different genetic, endotype, and biomarker patterns.

Translation of these data to clinical utility in the real world requires confirmation of consistency based on studies in large and diverse populations and the availability of practical and reliable testing methods that provide reproducible results. Nevertheless, there is strong research desire in AD to evolve to personalized medicine achieved through the accurate identification of specific phenotypes and endotypes of AD and through correlation with specific biomarker patterns [56–63]. Translation of these data to application in real-world clinical practice requires confirmation of consistency based on studies performed in large and diverse patient populations and the availability of practical, reliable, and cost-effective testing methods that provide reproducible results.

The development of personalized medicine in AD is a moving target at present but is progressing rapidly. One current issue requiring resolution is the lack of uniform and consistent use of AD phenotypes across multiple studies [57]. Some progress has been made in defining cytokine patterns in AD related to different phases of evolution; correlation of cytokine and biomarker patterns with different AD clinical presentations and endotypes such as age, race, and intrinsic/extrinsic subtypes; and fine-tuning treatment selection through identification of specific biomarker patterns and endotypes in AD [57, 58, 60, 62]. In one report, cluster analysis has identified four serum-based biomarker clusters in AD which could be predicted with a model using ten serum biomarkers and were distributed at different rates among study samples (cluster A [33.6%], skin-homing chemokines/IL-11R1 dominant; cluster B [18.5%], Th1/Th2/Th17 dominant; cluster C [18.5%], Th2/Th22/PARC-dominant; cluster D, [29.5%] Th2/eosinophil-inferior) [62]. Identification of well-defined cluster patterns based on biomarker measurement will hopefully lead to correlations with effective treatment selection. The International Eczema Council has subdivided potential biomarkers into categories based on their suggested clinical utility. These categories are biomarkers differentiating AD from psoriasis, biomarkers correlating with clinical AD severity, biomarkers that do not exhibit consistent correlation with AD severity, and biomarkers that can predict onset of AD and/or response to specific therapies [61]. Examples of predictive biomarker correlations reported in individual studies include dipeptidyl **peptidase**-4 (DPP-4) levels as a potential predictor of response to IL-13 inhibition for AD (tralokinumab), periostin levels as a possible IL-13 inhibition response biomarker in asthma, correlation of high baseline IL-22 levels in skin with response to fezakinumab in severe AD, and CXCL9 or CXCL2 level correlations with response to cyclosporine and dupilumab, respectively, for AD [61, 62, 64]. Personalized medicine and treatment practices are on their way and expected to move from the research benchtop to clinical dermatology clinics at some time in the relatively near future.

The development of tests that evaluate specific biomarker/cytokine patterns in AD or analyze genetic patterns of AD through transcriptomes obtained from skin biopsies or tape strips are likely to change how AD is managed over time. However, the practical incorporation of validated research tools that directly assess patient-reported outcome in clinical trials of AD subjects is very important to develop [65]. One such practical measure that is time-efficient and cost-effective for clinicians in practice that can be incorporated immediately is the Atopic Dermatitis Control Tool (ADCT) [66, 67]. This self-evaluation completed by the patient qualitatively and quantitatively assesses and grades how patients are affected by their AD throughout their entire day and the current level of AD control based on numerical responses given to six questions. The ADCT provides a more objective means of quantifying the current severity of AD for both the clinician and patient at any given point in time, thus facilitating discussion related to maintaining or changing their treatment. Completion and multiple visits allow for a documented blueprint of the course of the patient's AD and its response to treatments. The reader is referred to published literature on the ADCT for further details.

To conclude, what can we offer to our patient described in the case above to address her queries? New treatments for AD continue to emerge coupled with continued information on the pathophysiology of AD, both of which provide clinicians with an improved ability to treat AD more effectively. The development and availability of targeted therapies, especially monoclonal antibodies and JAK inhibitors, provide clinicians the ability to therapeutically manage flares of AD and effectively maintain suppression of both eczematous dermatitis and pruritus between major flares. Although personalized medicine and specific testing methods to help in selection of therapies and predict outcomes have not reached the point of routine availability in clinical practice, our patient can be encouraged that their availability may be coming soon as more research and development are performed. However, the ADCT may be incorporated into her management immediately and may assist in better following of her disease course and responses to treatment. Lastly, her decision whether or not to transition to an oral JAK inhibitor and discontinue monoclonal antibody use is a realistic consideration. Data are available on potential outcomes from this transition, along with what potential risks need to be considered and discussed and what follow-up and monitoring need to be completed over time.

**Board Review Question Explanation**

Which of the following binds to OX40L and prevents its interaction with OX40?

A. Dupilumab
B. Tralokinumab
C. Amlitelimab (correct)
D. Secukinumab
E. Ligelizumab

**Explanation**

Amlitelimab is a human non-depleting monoclonal antibody to OX40L that prevents binding interaction with OX40. This inhibition of OX40L binding to OX40 results in the blocking of antigen presenting cell-induced T cell activation and inhibits OX40L back signaling, thus aiming to restore immunologic homeostasis (pro-inflammatory and inflammatory T cell balance).

**Key Takeaway Points**

- The pathophysiology of atopic dermatitis (AD) is complex with an array of heterogenous clinical manifestations. Although upregulated Th2 inflammation is a major component of (AD) in many patients, there are a variety of several genetically defined endotypes which underscore the presence and relative magnitude of individual clinical manifestation of AD.
- Multiple systemic therapy options are currently available or in development for treatment of AD.
- Currently available FDA-approved systemic therapies include injectable monoclonal antibodies that inhibit both IL-4 and IL-13, or IL-13 alone, and oral Janus kinase (JAK) inhibitors that inhibit primarily JAK-1.
- Recommendations are available to guide clinical and laboratory monitoring in patients treated with a JAK inhibitor for AD.
- The pipeline for systemic management of AD addresses several potential modes of action which reflect the complex and heterogenous nature of AD that includes a broad range of clinical presentations affecting multiple age groups.
- Although not fully perfected to allow for routine clinical application at present, personalized medicine that incorporates genomic differentiation of subtypes (endotypes) of AD is expected to emerge over time and allow for more targeted approaches that can better address the therapeutic needs of the individual patient.

## References

1. Zuberbier T, Orlow SJ, Paller AS, et al. Patient perspectives on the management of atopic dermatitis. J Allergy Clin Immunol. 2006;118:226–32.
2. Paller AS, Siegfried EC, Vekeman F, et al. Treatment patterns of pediatric patients with atopic dermatitis: a claims data analysis. J Am Acad Dermatol. 2020;83:651–60.
3. Arzeno J, Hogeling M. Epidemiology. In: Chan L, Shi VY, editors. Atopic dermatitis: inside out or outside in? Philadelphia, PA: Elsevier; 2023. p. 25–33.
4. Abuabara K, Margolis DJ, Langan M. The long-term course of atopic dermatitis. Dermatol Clin. 2017;35:291–7.
5. Bieber T. How to define atopic dermatitis? Dermatol Clin. 2017;35:275–81.
6. Chan L. Atopy of the skin. In: Chan L, Shi VY, editors. Atopic dermatitis: inside out or outside in? Philadelphia, PA: Elsevier; 2023. p. 17–24.
7. Li H, Zhang Z, Zhang H, et al. Update on the pathogenesis and therapy of atopic dermatitis. Clin Rev Allergy Immunol. 2021;61(3):324–38.
8. Kim J, Kim BE, Leung DYM. Pathophysiology of atopic dermatitis: clinical implications. Allergy Asthma Proc. 2019;40(2):84–92.
9. Hanifin J. Adult-onset atopic dermatitis: fact or fancy? Dermatol Clin. 2017;35:299–302.
10. Boguniewicz M, Fonacier L, Guttman-Yassky E, et al. Atopic dermatitis yardstick: practical recommendations for an evolving therapeutic landscape. Ann Allergy Asthma Immunol. 2018;120:10–22.

11. Puar N, Chovatiya R, Paller AS. New treatments in atopic dermatitis. Ann Allergy Asthma Immunol. 2021;126(1):21–31.
12. Prezzano JC, Beck LA. Long-term treatment of atopic dermatitis. Dermatol Clin. 2017;35:335–49.
13. Zhou S, Qi F, Gong Y, et al. Biological therapies for atopic dermatitis: a systematic review. Dermatology. 2021;237(4):542–52.
14. Yamamura K, Nakahara T. The dawn of a new era in atopic dermatitis treatment. J Clin Med. 2022;11(20):6145.
15. Scott JB, Paller AS. Novel treatments for pediatric atopic dermatitis. Curr Opin Pediatr. 2021;33(4):392–401.
16. Paller AS, Siegfried EC, Thaçi D, et al. Efficacy and safety of dupilumab with concomitant topical corticosteroids in children 6 to 11 years old with severe atopic dermatitis: a randomized, double-blinded, placebo-controlled phase 3 trial. J Am Acad Dermatol. 2020;83(5):1282–93.
17. Del Rosso JQ. Monoclonal antibody therapies for atopic dermatitis: where are we now in the spectrum of disease management? J Clin Aesthet Dermatol. 2019;12(2):39–41.
18. Deleuran M, Thaçi D, Beck LA, et al. Dupilumab shows long-term safety and efficacy in patients with moderate to severe atopic dermatitis enrolled in a phase 3 open-label extension study. J Am Acad Dermatol. 2020;82(2):377–88.
19. Wollenberg A, Blauvelt A, Guttman-Yassky E, et al. Tralokinumab for moderate-to-severe atopic dermatitis: results from two 52-week, randomized, double-blind, multicenter, placebo-controlled phase III trials (ECZTRA 1 and ECZTRA 2). Br J Dermatol. 2021;184(3):437–49.
20. Nezamololama N, Fieldhouse K, Metzger K, Gooderham M. Emerging systemic JAK inhibitors in the treatment of atopic dermatitis: a review of abrocitinib, baricitinib, and upadacitinib. Drugs Context. 2020;9:2020-8-5.
21. Chovatiya R, Paller AS. JAK inhibitors in the treatment of atopic dermatitis. J Allergy Clin Immunol. 2021;148(4):927–40.
22. Papp K, Szepietowski JC, Kircik L, et al. Efficacy and safety of ruxolitinib cream for the treatment of atopic dermatitis: results from 2 phase 3, randomized, double-blind studies. J Am Acad Dermatol. 2021;85(4):863–72.
23. Gong X, Chen X, Kuligowski ME, et al. Pharmacokinetics of ruxolitinib in patients with atopic dermatitis treated with ruxolitinib cream: data from phase II and III studies. Am J Clin Dermatol. 2021;22(4):555–66.
24. Pezzolo E, Naldi L. Tralokinumab in the treatment of resistant atopic dermatitis: an open-label, retrospective case series study. JEADV. 2022; https://doi.org/10.1111/jdv.18753.
25. Silverberg J, Thyssen JP, Fahrbach K, et al. Comparative efficacy and safety of systemic therapies used in moderate-to-severe atopic dermatitis: a systematic literature review and network meta-analysis. J Eur Acad Dermatol Venereol. 2021;35(9):1797–810.
26. Abrocitinib tablets for oral use (CIBINQO), Prescribing information, Pfizer labs (division of Pfizer Inc, New York, NY; 2022.
27. Upadacitinib extended-release tablets for oral use (RINVOQ), Prescribing information, AbbVie Biotechnology Ltd, AbbVie Inc, North Chicago, IL; 2019.
28. Blauvelt A, Teixeira HD, Simpson EL, et al. Efficacy and safety of upadacitinib vs dupilumab in adults with moderate-to-severe atopic dermatitis: a randomized clinical trial. JAMA Dermatol. 2021;157(9):1047–55.
29. Bieber T, Simpson EL, Silverberg J, et al. Comparing abrocitinib and dupilumab in the treatment of atopic dermatitis: a plain language summary. Immunotherapy. 2022;14(1):5–14.
30. Silverberg JS, Simpson EL, Thyssen JP, et al. Switching from dupilumab to abrocitinib in patients with moderate-to-severe atopic dermatitis; an analysis of responders and non-responders to dupilumab. Presented at the Revolutionizing Atopic Dermatitis (RAD) virtual conference, December 11; 2022.
31. Slomski A. Oral upadacitinib beats subcutaneous dupilumab for atopic dermatitis. JAMA. 2021;326(13):1246.

32. Nash P, Kerschbaumer A, Dörner T, et al. Points to consider for the treatment of immune-mediated inflammatory diseases with Janus kinase inhibitors: a consensus statement. Ann Rheum Dis. 2021;80:71–87.
33. Simpson ES, Papp KA, Blauvelt A, et al. Efficacy and safety of upadacitinib in patients with moderate to severe atopic dermatitis: analysis of follow-up data from the measure up 1 and measure up 2 randomized clinical trials. JAMA Dermatol. 2022;158(4):404–13.
34. Kristian Reich K, Thyssen JP, Blauvelt A, et al. Efficacy and safety of abrocitinib versus dupilumab in adults with moderate-to-severe atopic dermatitis: a randomized, double-blind, multicenter phase 3 trial. Lancet. 2022;400(10348):273–82.
35. King B, Ohyama M, Kwon O, et al. Two phase 3 trials of baricitinib for alopecia areata. N Engl J Med. 2022;386(18):1687–99.
36. Kwon O, Senna MM, Sinclair R, et al. Long-term efficacy and safety of baricitinib in patients with severe alopecia areata: week 52 results from BRAVE-AA1 and BRAVE-AA2. Poster presented at Winter Clinical Miami, Miami, FL, USA, February 17-20, 2023.
37. Tai-Li Chen TL, Lee LL, Huang HK, et al. Association of risk of incident venous thromboembolism with atopic dermatitis and treatment with Janus kinase inhibitors: a systematic review and meta-analysis. JAMA Dermatol. 2022;158(11):1254–61.
38. Daniele S, Bunick C. JAK inhibitor safety compared to traditional systemic immunosuppressive therapies. J Drugs Dermatol. 2022;21(12):1298–303.
39. Yang N, Chen Z, Zhang X, Shi Y. Novel targeted biological agents for the treatment of atopic dermatitis. BioDrugs. 2021;35(4):401–15.
40. Del Rosso JQ. More from the pipeline of clinical research on selected systemic therapies for atopic dermatitis. J Clin Aesthet Dermatol. 2019;12(5):49–53.
41. Ultsch M, Bevers J, Nakamura G, et al. Structural basis of signaling blockade by anti-IL-13 antibody lebrikizumab. J Mol Biol. 2013;425(8):1330–9.
42. Guttman-Yassky E, Blauvelt A, Eichenfield LF, et al. Efficacy and safety of lebrikizumab, a high-affinity interleukin 13 inhibitor, in adults with moderate to severe atopic dermatitis: a phase 2b randomized clinical trial. JAMA Dermatol. 2020;156(4):411–20.
43. Simpson E, Gooderham M, Wollenberg A, et al. Efficacy and safety of lebrikizumab in combination with topical corticosteroids in adolescents and adults with moderate-to-severe atopic dermatitis: a randomized clinical trial (ADhere). JAMA Dermatol. 2023; https://doi.org/10.1001/jamadermatol.2022.5534. Online ahead of print.
44. Blauvelt A, et al. Poster presentation. Fall Clinical Dermatology, Las Vegas, NV, October 2022.
45. Labib A, Vander Does A, Yosipovitch G. Nemolizumab for atopic dermatitis. Drugs Today (Barc). 2022;58(4):159–73.
46. Kabashima K, Matsumura T, Komazaki H, et al. Trial of nemolizumab and topical agents for atopic dermatitis with pruritus. N Engl J Med. 2020;383(2):141–50.
47. Ratchataswan T, Banzon TM, Thyssen JP, et al. Biologics for treatment of atopic dermatitis: current status and future prospect. J Allergy Clin Immunol Pract. 2021;9(3):1053–65.
48. Lee GR, Lee DE, Shi VY. Emerging targeted treatments. In: Chan L, Shi VY, editors. Atopic dermatitis: inside out or outside in? Philadelphia, PA: Elsevier; 2023. p. 237–51.
49. Furue M, Furue M. OX-40L-OX40 signaling in atopic dermatitis. J Clin Med. 2021;10:2578. https://doi.org/10.3390/jcm10122578.
50. Webb GW, Hirschfield GM, Lane PJL. OX40, OX40L and autoimmunity: a comprehensive review. Clin Rev Allergy Immunol. 2016;50:312–32.
51. Le AM, Torre T. OX40-OX40L inhibition for the treatment of atopic dermatitis-focus on rocatinlimab and amlitelimab. Pharmaceutics. 2022;14:2753. https://doi.org/10.3390/pharmaceutics14122753.
52. Weidinger S, Michael Cork, Reich A, et al. Amlitelimab reduces serum IL-13 in a Phase 2a clinical trial in atopic dermatitis without impacting T-cell expansion in a T-cell recall assay. Poster presented at the Revolutionizing Atopic Dermatitis Virtual Conference, December 11, 2022.

53. Simpson EL, Parnes JR, She D, et al. Tezepelumab, an anti-thymic stromal lymphopoietin monoclonal antibody, in the treatment of moderate to severe atopic dermatitis: a randomized phase 2a clinical trial. J Am Acad Dermatol. 2019;80(4):1013–21.
54. Chan S, Cornelius V, Cro S, et al. Treatment effect of omalizumab on severe pediatric atopic dermatitis: the ADAPT randomized clinical trial. JAMA Pediatr. 2020;174(1):29–37.
55. Sugaya M. The role of Th17-related cytokines in atopic dermatitis. Int J Molec Sci. 2020;21:1314.
56. Cabanillas B, Brehler AC, Novak N. Atopic dermatitis phenotypes and the need for personalized medicine. Curr Opin Allergy. 2017;17(4):309–15.
57. Bosma A, Ascott A, Iskandar R, et al. Classifying atopic dermatitis: a systematic review of phenotypes and associated characteristics. JEADV. 2022;36:807–19.
58. Patruno C, Potestio L, Napolitano M. Clinical phenotypes of adult atopic dermatitis and related therapies. Curr Opin Allergy Clin Immunol. 2022;22(4):242–9.
59. Hassan S, Hamideh N, Poulos C, et al. Atopic dermatitis biomarkers and the movement toward personalized treatment. Dermatitis. 2021;32(1S):S8–14.
60. Fania L, Moretta G, Antonelli F, et al. Multiple roles for cytokines in atopic dermatitis: from pathogenic mediators to endotype-specific biomarkers to therapeutic targets. Int J Molec Sci. 2022;23:2684. https://doi.org/10.3390/ijms23052684.
61. Yael R-Y, Thyssen JP, Bissonnette R, et al. Biomarkers in atopic dermatitis—a review on behalf of the international eczema council. J Allergy Clin Immunol. 2021;147(4):1174–90.
62. Bakker DS, Nierkens S, Knol EF, et al. Confirmation of multiple endotypes in atopic dermatitis based on serum biomarkers. J Allergy Clin Immunol. 2021;147(1):189–98.
63. Andersson AM, Solberg J, Koch A, et al. Assessment of biomarkers in pediatric atopic dermatitis by tape strips and skin biopsies. Allergy. 2022;77(5):1499–509.
64. Glickman JW, Han J, Garcet S, et al. Improving evaluation of drugs in atopic dermatitis by combining clinical and molecular measures. J Allergy Clin Immunol. 2020;8:3622–3625.e19.
65. Silverberg J, Margolis DJ, Boguniewicz M, et al. Validation of five patient-reported outcomes for atopic dermatitis severity in adults. Br J Dermatol. 2020;182(1):104–11.
66. Kido-Nakahara M, Yokote G, Yoshida M, et al. Atopic dermatitis control tool (ADCT): a useful tool for self-evaluation in patients with atopic dermatitis. J Dermatol. 2021;48(12):1951–2.
67. Staumont-Sallé D, Taieb C, Merhand S, Shourick S. The atopic dermatitis control tool: a high-performance tool for optimal support. Acta Derm Venereol. 2021;101(12) https://doi.org/10.2340/actadv.v101.750.

# Chapter 21
# Comorbidities of AD

**Janell Tully and Daniel C. Butler**

**Case Title** A 68-year-old biology professor with atopic dermatitis and new onset dysphagia presents for follow-up at the dermatologist.

**Case**
It is a Tuesday afternoon in the dermatology clinic, and Mr. E, a friendly 68-year-old male biology professor with a history of cardiovascular disease and a recent diagnosis of atopic dermatitis in the past 2 years, presents for follow-up. He notes that while growing up he had asthma and hay fever but otherwise was healthy. Although his AD remains well-controlled today, he mentions that he meets with his primary care physician next week to discuss new-onset heartburn that does not improve with antacids and the "feeling of food getting stuck in his throat." Mr. E shares that he is curious whether his conditions may be related and asks to learn more in depth about the comorbid conditions associated with atopic dermatitis.

**Board Review Question**
What is an important etiology to consider in a young male patient with atopic dermatitis who complains of indigestion and dysphagia?

A. Malignancy
B. Eosinophilic esophagitis
C. Gastroesophageal reflux disease (GERD)
D. Scleroderma
E. Achalasia

J. Tully
University of Arizona College of Medicine—Phoenix, Phoenix, AZ, USA
e-mail: janelltully@email.arizona.edu

D. C. Butler (✉)
University of Arizona College of Medicine- Tucson, Tucson, AZ, USA
e-mail: dcbutler@arizona.edu



N. Brownstone et al. (eds.), *Clinical Cases in Atopic Dermatitis*, Clinical Cases in Dermatology, https://doi.org/10.1007/978-3-031-52147-8_21

# Main Text

## Introduction

Derived from the Ancient Greek word *atopía* meaning "without place," the term *atopy* was used by Arthur Coca and Robert Cooke in the early 1920s to group together the inheritable abnormal non-anaphylactic hypersensitivity responses observed in patients with asthma and allergic rhinitis [1, 2]. Atopic dermatitis (AD) would be described in the following decade and later recognized by Coca and colleagues as another hypersensitivity condition related to atopy [1]. Today, atopy (and, therefore, atopic disease) is recognized as the predisposition to develop exaggerated immune responses to antigens or allergens characterized by CD4+ Th2 differentiation and the overproduction of immunoglobulin E (IgE) [3].

The most common atopic diseases include allergic rhinitis, allergic asthma, AD, and food allergies [3]. Epidemiological studies have demonstrated that these allergic diseases may co-occur and present in a sequential manner beginning with the manifestation of AD early in life followed later by the development of allergic rhinitis and asthma [4, 5]. This phenomenon is referred to as the "atopic march." While some support the temporal nature of the atopic march, others have suggested that this may be an oversimplification of complex genetic and environmental interactions resulting in multimorbidity of atopic diseases [4–6]. Nevertheless, the impact of AD often extends far beyond its negative impact on the skin, and individuals with AD experience increased rates of comorbid conditions. In this chapter we will discuss common comorbidities of AD and highlight the possible systemic impacts of AD through emerging associations with non-allergic comorbid disease.

## Section 1: Allergic Comorbidities (Table 21.1)

### Asthma and Allergic Rhinitis

Cross-sectional, case-control, and cohort studies have consistently shown that asthma is common among patients with AD [7–9]. In a systematic review and meta-analysis, Ravnborg and colleagues found that among 67 observational studies, there was a significant association between AD and asthma even when controlling for physician-diagnosed disease (pooled OR, 3.03; 95% CI, 2.64–3.47) [7]. They also found no significant variation in association when studies were divided by age, disease activity, or study design [7]. A systemic review of 13 prospective cohort studies (four birth cohort studies and nine eczema cohort studies) had similar findings, although the risk of developing asthma in the setting of atopic eczema was slightly lower (pooled OR, 2.14; 95% CI, 1.67–2.75) [10].

Multiple risk factors for the development of asthma in patients with AD have been identified, including IgE sensitization and filaggrin deficiency [8]. AD severity

**Table 21.1** Allergic comorbidities in atopic dermatitis key points

| Comorbidity | Estimated prevalence | Estimated risk | Key point | Therapeutic considerations |
|---|---|---|---|---|
| Asthma [7, 11, 18] | 25% | Children: 2.78 (95% CI, 2.50–3.10)[a] Adults: 1.68 (95% CI, 1.48–1.80)[b] | Increasing AD severity is associated with an increased risk of developing asthma | Consider a therapy that targets both conditions, such as dupilumab |
| Allergic rhinitis [12, 16–19, 62] | 1%–39% | Children: 4.53 (95% CI, 2.13–9.63)[b] Adults: 1.55 (95% CI, 1.31–1.84)[a] | Having more than one component of the atopic triad has been associated with poorer AD control | Sedating antihistamines may provide a dual benefit for allergic rhinitis symptoms and sleeping difficulties due to pruritus caused by AD |
| Food allergy [18, 23, 28, 39, 40] | 11%–30% | Children:[c] 2.30 (95% CI, 1.60–3.50)[a] Adults: 2.45 (95% CI, 1.79–3.06)[b] | Epicutaneous sensitization through an impaired skin barrier can result in a clinical food allergy | Skin barrier repair and broader AD management may help prevent epicutaneous sensitization Allergen avoidance is key in patients with IgE-mediated allergies, but the risks and benefits of elimination diets to improve AD should otherwise be carefully considered |
| Eosinophilic esophagitis (EoE) [18, 54–56, 59–61] | 2–46% | Children: 3.10 (95% CI, 2.40–4.00)[a] Adults: 1.53 (95% CI, 1.47–1.60)[b] | If young male with AD and GI symptoms, consider a workup for EoE | Consider the role anti-IL-13 biologics, such as dupilumab, in treating both conditions |

*AD* Atopic dermatitis, *IgE* Immunoglobulin-E, *GI* Gastrointestinal, *IL-13* Interleukin-13
[a]Odds ratio
[b]Relative risk
[c]Personal history of atopic dermatitis in the first 2 years of life

has also been significantly associated with the appearance of asthma later in childhood [11]. In a study of 205 children with AD, those with moderate and severe AD were at greater risk for the onset of asthma in the first 4 years of life as compared to individuals with mild AD (moderate AD, $p = 0.032$; severe AD, $p = 0.0001$) [11]. However, there are conflicting findings; one meta-analysis found no significant difference of pooled prevalence based on mild versus moderate to severe AD or by current AD vs ever AD [7].

Like asthma, allergic rhinitis is common among children with AD; Kapoor et al. found that nearly 38% of children with physician-confirmed AD reported symptoms of both asthma and allergic rhinitis by 3 years of age [12]. Allergic rhinitis is characterized by sneezing, nasal congestion, rhinorrhea, and/or nasal pruritus caused by an allergic response to inhaled antigens. The response occurs in two phases: an early IgE-mediated phase driven by Th2 immune cell activation and a late phase comprised of an influx of cytokines, including interleukins (IL)-4 and IL-13 [13]. Although highly prevalent in the general population [13], individuals with AD may be at an increased risk for developing allergic rhinitis, especially those with early-onset or more severe AD [4, 9, 14].

In a prospective, longitudinal Swedish cohort study, eczema in the first year of life was identified as an independent risk factor for allergic rhinitis at 4.5 years of age (OR, 1.97; 95% CI, 1.19–3.26; $p = 0.009$) [15]. These findings are consistent with a longitudinal study of over 2000 children, which found that the presence of AD at 1 year was associated with more than a fourfold increased risk of allergic rhinitis at 3 years of age (RR, 4.53; 95% CI, 2.13–9.63) [16]. In this same study, allergic sensitization in the setting of AD increased the risk of allergic rhinitis more than 11-fold (adjusted RR, 11.75; 95% CI, 5.73–24.12) [16]. Interestingly, AD without allergic sensitization was not associated with an increased risk of asthma compared to non-sensitized children without AD (adjusted RR, 0.46; 95% CI, 0.011–1.93). However, children with AD and allergic sensitization had a sevenfold increased risk for asthma (adjusted RR, 7.04; 95% CI, 4.13–11.99) [16].

Individuals with early onset of more than one component of the atopic triad (AD, asthma, or allergic rhinitis) have been shown to have worse disease control, and individuals with both asthma and AD in childhood may indicate the presence of a more persistent AD phenotype [12, 17]. When managing a patient with concurrent AD and asthma, choosing a therapy that targets both conditions, such as dupilumab, can be beneficial [18]. Additionally, although oral antihistamines have not consistently shown efficacy in managing symptoms of AD in clinical trials, they can provide relief for patients with who have concurrent allergic rhinitis, and sedating oral antihistamines may provide a dual benefit for patients who experience difficulty sleeping due to pruritus [19].

## Food Sensitization and Food Allergy

The relationship between food sensitization, food allergy, and atopic dermatitis is well-established [20, 21]. A cornerstone of AD is skin barrier dysfunction, which not only contributes to skin inflammation but may also allow potential allergens to penetrate the skin, consequently resulting in food sensitization (epicutaneous sensitization) and potentially a clinically relevant food allergy [22–25]. Therefore, although food sensitization in the first few years of life and the presence of a food allergy in adolescence have been associated with an increased risk of developing AD [26–28], food allergy may also follow the development of AD [20, 29, 30]. Intriguingly, while epicutaneous sensitization through an impaired skin barrier results in cytokine dysregulation and can ultimately provoke a clinical food allergy, early oral food allergen exposure is likely protective [24]. Furthermore, multiple studies have demonstrated that delaying solid food introduction, and, therefore, possible oral allergens, is neither associated with decreased food sensitization nor the development of food allergies or atopic dermatitis [31, 32].

There are three primary endotypes of food allergy: IgE-mediated (immediate type hypersensitivity), non-IgE mediated (delayed type hypersensitivity), and mixed (IgE/non-IgE) food allergy [33]. All three food allergy endotypes have been linked to AD [20, 34]; however non-IgE mediated and mixed food allergies remain less established [35]. Furthermore, although there is clear and strong evidence linking food allergy with AD, the heterogeneity of study methods (e.g., food allergens studied, definition of food allergy, and method used to establish presence or absence of allergy, such as physician diagnosis vs self-report) has made it difficult to estimate the true prevalence and clinical implications of food allergy among patients with AD [18]. The prevalence of food allergy among patients with AD ranges widely between studies and has been reported to be as high as 80% [20, 36]. However, in a pooled prevalence of seven studies estimated, the overall prevalence of food allergy among adults with AD is 11.2% (95% CI, 6–16.4%; $p < 0.001$) [18].

AD severity appears to play a role in the relationship between AD and IgE-mediated food allergy [37, 38]. One cross-sectional US adult population-based study found that increasing AD severity was associated with an increasing risk of food allergy where mild AD was associated with a mild but significant risk of food allergy (adjusted RR, 1.48; $p = 0.08$), whereas severe AD was associated with a much larger risk (adjusted RR, 8.49; $p < 0.0001$) [38]. The prevalence of IgE-mediated food allergy to top six allergens (milk, egg, wheat, soy, peanut, and fish) has been reported to be as high as 30% among children with moderate-to-severe AD [39].

The diagnosis for IgE-mediated food allergies is typically straightforward and can be often made through a convincing history, which is less reliable among non-IgE (delayed) food allergies [40]. Currently, the gold standard for diagnosing a food allergy is a Double-Blind, Placebo-Controlled Food Challenge (DBPCFC) [40–42]. Notably, there are cases of IgE-mediated allergies that also result in late eczematous reactions, and therefore, the methods used for a DBPCFC should extend multiple days to capture these reactions [41]. When a DBPCFC is unavailable or cost prohibitive, both food-specific immunoglobulins E (SpIgE) and the skin prick test (SPT) may also be used to help identify IgE-mediated food allergies [40, 43]. Alternatively, patch testing has been proposed to assess for non-IgE mediated or mixed food allergies by directly applying food extract to the patient's skin, but conflicting results about its diagnostic value have been reported, which may be related to its non-standardized methods [40, 44]. The American Academy of Allergy, Asthma, and Immunology (AAAAI) Allergic Skin Diseases Committee recently published a comprehensive review of AD and food allergy, in which they recommended evaluating for milk, egg, peanut, wheat, and soy sensitization if a patient is less than 5 years of age [45].

Recommendations for the therapeutic management for patients with AD and concurrent food allergy vary greatly. Food avoidance is key for IgE-mediated reactions, which may otherwise progress to life-threatening anaphylactic reactions [40]. Conversely, food elimination among patients with non-IgE mediated allergies or who have food-triggered AD is more controversial [45]. Some cite that elimination may result in lost tolerance and that patients with food-triggered AD have been documented to develop IgE-mediated allergy on re-exposure [46]. Thus, food elimination in these cases should be thoughtfully considered, and the benefits of AD improvement should be weighed against the potential for the potential harms of elimination diets, which also include nutritional deficiency, cost and difficulty implementing the diet, and/or associated anxiety [20, 44]. Regardless of dietary changes, the role of skin barrier dysfunction in allergen sensitization emphasizes the critical role of skin barrier repair and broader AD management [21, 23, 40, 45, 47]. Nevertheless, several studies have sought (and continue to seek) to understand the role of food allergy screening among patients with AD, which has been cited as one of the highest priority research questions for AD [18, 48, 49].

## Eosinophilic Esophagitis

Eosinophilic esophagitis (EoE) is an antigen-mediated inflammatory disease characterized by eosinophilic infiltration into the esophageal mucosa leading to esophageal dysfunction [50, 51]. In children, this typically first presents as food aversion, poor appetite, vomiting, and/or abdominal pain [52]. Adolescents and adults with EoE are more likely to complain of dysphagia with or without food impaction [50, 52]. Although rare, there are multiple other conditions associated with esophageal eosinophilia and dysphagia, such as parasitic infections, allergic vasculitis, Crohn's disease, and drug hypersensitivity [50, 53]. Instead, EoE is increasingly recognized as an allergic disorder that can occur concomitantly with AD in adults and other atopic conditions [51, 54].

The estimated prevalence of AD among patients with EoE ranges between 2% and 19% with one study reporting the prevalence of comorbid AD and EoE as high as 46.1% [54, 55]. Moreover, children with EoE have significantly higher odds of also having AD as compared to children without EoE (OR, 3.1; 95% CI, 2.4–4.0; $p < 0.0001$) [56]. Interestingly, as seen in the atopic march, an AD diagnosis also typically precedes a diagnosis of EoE; in a retrospective administrative database analysis of patients in the United States between 2009 and 2013, AD was diagnosed, on average, roughly 6 months prior to EoE (mean days prior to EoE diagnosis ± standard error, −169.4 ± 14.8; 95% CI, −140.2 to −198.5 days) [54].

Among 77 patients, ages 3–21 years, with EoE, Daley et al. [57] found that patients with EoE and AD (versus EoE without AD) had significantly higher eosinophil counts in the esophagus (65 eos/hpf vs 40 eos/hpf, respectively; $p = 0.005$). However, there were no significant differences in the presence of subepithelial fibrosis, esophageal strictures, the presence of microabscesses, or food impaction [57]. Nevertheless, the histopathologic abnormalities and symptoms of EoE can extend beyond the esophagus to other segments of the gastrointestinal (GI) tract [52]. Therefore, children with AD who present with GI symptoms should be evaluated for concurrent EoE, especially if they are male, as multiple studies have found that EoE more commonly affects males than females [50, 52, 56].

Like AD, EoE is characterized by Th2 predominant inflammation and the production of Th2-related cytokines, including IL-13 [58]. Multiple studies evaluating the role of anti-IL-13 monoclonal antibodies in the treatment of EoE have shown promising results [59–61]. One multicenter, randomized, double-blind, parallel-group, placebo-controlled phase 2 study evaluated the efficacy and safety of dupilumab in the treatment of patients with active EoE. In this study, they found dupilumab to be well-tolerated, reduce dysphagia, and improve the histologic and endoscopic features of EoE [60]. Although further research is needed to evaluate the role of dupilumab in treating patients with both EoE and AD, these results highlight the value of selecting therapies that may derive multiple benefits for certain patients.

## *Section 2: Emerging Data on Multimorbidity Among Patients with Atopic Dermatitis*

Given the rising prevalence of AD; its impact on physical, psychological, and social well-being; and its heterogeneity in presentation, increasing attention is being given to non-allergic comorbidities. These include possible systemic conditions including obesity, bone health, and cardiovascular disease.

### Obesity

Although typically recognized simply as excess body weight for a given height, obesity is a complex and multifactorial disease that currently affects over one-third of the global population [63]. Obesity is associated with increased risk and morbidity of numerous chronic conditions, including type II diabetes, cardiovascular disease, and depression [63]. Obesity and asthma also frequently co-occur, and a possible bidirectional relationship between the two has been identified [64–66]. Given the well-established role of atopy in the development of asthma, greater attention has been given recently to the possible relationship between obesity and atopy, including atopic dermatitis [65].

Multiple studies have found a positive association between obesity and AD [67–72]. Interestingly, Silverberg et al. found that obesity was significantly associated with increased AD in adults [71] but was only significantly associated with AD in children when obesity started prior to age 5 years and was present for more than 2.5 years [72]. These findings are consistent with a longitudinal birth cohort study of 731 children that found increased BMI significantly increased the risk of physician-diagnosed eczema at ages 5 (OR, 1.23; 95% CI, 1.04–1.47; $p = 0.02$) and 8 years (OR, 1.23; 95% CI, 1.03–1.45; $p = 0.02$) [69].

Conversely, other studies have reported no significant associations between obesity and AD [68, 73, 74]. Moreover, in a cross-sectional analysis of adults with atopic eczema, while having mild or moderate atopic eczema was associated with significantly higher odds of being overweight or obese (7% and 15% increased odds, respectively), there was no association between being overweight/obese and having severe atopic eczema (adjusted OR, 1.00; 95% CI, 0.96–1.03) [67].

## Bone Health

Characterized by chronic and relapsing skin inflammation, and increasingly recognized as a systemic inflammatory disorder [75], there is strong evidence suggesting that AD is associated with impaired bone health [18]. Chronic systemic inflammation can alter bone metabolism resulting in increased bone resorption and bone loss [76]. Similar aberrations in bone metabolism are seen in chronic skin inflammation, which may be mediated by IL-17 (a pro-inflammatory cytokine produced by Th17 cells) inhibition of Wnt signaling in osteoblasts (bone building cells) [77, 78]. In AD, filaggrin deficiency may drive increased production of peripheral Th17 cells [79].

Multiple studies have linked AD with an increased risk of developing osteoporosis [80–82]. In a meta-analysis comprised of more than 105 million participants, patients with AD had much higher odds of having osteoporosis compared to those without AD (OR, 1.95; 95% CI, 1.18–3.23; $p = 0.009$) [83]. Other studies have also identified that AD is associated with an increased risk of fracture [80, 84, 85] and that the risk of osteoporosis-related fractures among patients with severe AD is significantly higher (OR, 1.13; 95% CI, 1.05–1.22; $p = 0.001$) [83]. In addition to the increased risk of impaired bone health due to systemic inflammation, chronic oral, and possibly potent topical, corticosteroid use is associated with increased fracture risk [86, 87]. Accordingly, additional research on how to reduce the risk of bone loss and fractures among patients with AD is needed [86], including the potential role for guidelines to identify candidates for fracture prevention therapy [18].

## Cardiovascular Disease

Skin inflammation has been linked to vascular inflammation [88], and multiple inflammatory skin diseases have been associated with increased cardiovascular (CV) risk [89]. Multiple studies have looked at the possible relationship between AD and cardiovascular disease (CVD) [18]. In a systemic review and meta-analysis, Ascott et al. found no overall association between AD and CV outcomes but did find a mean relative risk increase of 1.15 (95% CI, 1.09–1.21) for any CV outcome (angina, CV death, heart failure, ischemic stroke, stroke, and/or myocardial infarction) [90]. Another systematic review and meta-analysis found that although mild AD was not associated with hypertension, both moderate and severe AD were associated with increases in hypertension as compared to healthy adult controls (pooled prevalence 24.9% vs 14.7%, respectively; OR, 2.33; 95% CI, 1.10–4.94) [91].

In a recent guideline released by the American Academy of Dermatology on the "Awareness of comorbidities associated with atopic dermatitis in adults," the authors indicate that although there is moderate evidence to suggest that AD is likely to be associated with coronary artery disease, peripheral artery disease, and hypertension, the absolute risk of CVD attributable to AD remains small. They also point to the need for further research to establish whether treating AD reduces the risks of CVD [18]. Drucker and Harvey also highlight the current limitations in data on the role of AD management in reducing CV risk, but do note that improving AD may also improve patient sleep, mood, and exercise tolerability, which, in turn, could decrease overall CV risk [92].

## *Summary*

Atopic dermatitis is characterized by chronic, relapsing skin inflammation though its negative impacts often extend beyond the skin. AD is increasingly recognized as a systemic disorder and has been associated with multiple comorbidities. As demonstrated in the atopic march, AD significantly increases the risk for developing other allergic conditions, such as asthma, allergic rhinitis, and food allergy [9, 24]. In recent years, AD has also been linked to eosinophilic esophagitis, a Th2 predominant inflammatory disorder of the esophagus [50, 54, 55].

In addition to the well-established allergic comorbidities of AD discussed here, there is evidence that suggests AD is also likely associated with obesity, impaired bone health, and increased cardiovascular risk [18]. While several mechanisms have been proposed to help explain the relationship between AD and its comorbidities, skin barrier dysfunction and inflammation may play key roles in driving some of these relationships [93, 94]. Collectively, the multimorbidity of AD emphasizes the need to address its systemic nature in comorbidity recognition and therapeutic management targeted at both symptom improvement and possible comorbidity prevention.

**Board Review Question Explanation**

What is an important etiology to consider in a young male patient with atopic dermatitis who complains of indigestion and dysphagia?

A. Malignancy
B. Eosinophilic esophagitis (correct)
C. Gastroesophageal reflux disease (GERD)
D. Scleroderma
E. Achalasia

**Explanation**

A. Incorrect. Although indigestion and dysphagia could be caused by malignancy, this is less likely in a young patient and in the absence of other symptoms, such as weight loss.
B. Correct. Eosinophilic esophagitis (EoE) is a Th2 predominant inflammatory disorder of the esophagus leading to esophageal dysfunction, which is characterized clinically by dysphagia and indigestion [52, 58]. EoE is more common in males than females and should be considered in young patients with AD who present with gastrointestinal symptoms [52].
C. Incorrect. Although a common cause of indigestion and dysphagia, eosinophilic esophagitis is an important etiology to consider in a young patient with atopic dermatitis.
D. Incorrect. Scleroderma has been associated with AD in female patients [95] and is less likely the diagnosis in this male patient with dysphagia.
E. Incorrect. Achalasia is an uncommon cause of dysphagia and is less likely the cause of dysphagia than EoE in a young patient with atopic dermatitis.

**Key Takeaway Points**

- Atopic dermatitis has been associated with several comorbid conditions, such as asthma, allergic rhinitis, eosinophilic esophagitis, food allergy, obesity, impaired bone health, and cardiovascular disease.
- Increasing atopic dermatitis severity appears to play a significant role in increasing prevalence of certain comorbid conditions, including asthma, allergic rhinitis, and IgE-mediated food allergy.
- Clinicians should use the presence of comorbidities to drive therapeutic decisions and to aid optimizing treatment adherence in patients with atopic dermatitis.

## References

1. Kramer ON, Strom MA, Ladizinski B, Lio PA. The history of atopic dermatitis. Clin Dermatol. 2017;35(4):344–8.
2. Coca AF, Cooke RA. On the classification of the phenomena of hypersensitiveness. J Immunol. 1923;8(3):163–82.
3. Justiz Vaillant AA, Modi P, Jan A. Atopy. StatPearls. Treasure Island (FL): StatPearls Publishing Copyright © 2022, StatPearls Publishing LLC.; 2022.
4. Yang L, Fu J, Zhou Y. Research progress in atopic march. Front Immunol. 2020;11:1907.
5. Khan SJ, Dharmage SC, Matheson MC, Gurrin LC. Is the atopic march related to confounding by genetics and early-life environment? A systematic review of sibship and twin data. Allergy. 2018;73(1):17–28.
6. Bantz SK, Zhu Z, Zheng T. The atopic march: progression from atopic dermatitis to allergic rhinitis and asthma. J Clin Cell Immunol. 2014;5(2)
7. Ravnborg N, Ambikaibalan D, Agnihotri G, Price S, Rastogi S, Patel KR, et al. Prevalence of asthma in patients with atopic dermatitis: a systematic review and meta-analysis. J Am Acad Dermatol. 2021;84(2):471–8.
8. Simpson EL. Comorbidity in atopic dermatitis. Curr Dermatol Rep. 2012;1(1):29–38.

9. von Kobyletzki LB, Bornehag CG, Hasselgren M, Larsson M, Lindström CB, Svensson Å. Eczema in early childhood is strongly associated with the development of asthma and rhinitis in a prospective cohort. BMC Dermatol. 2012;12:11.
10. van der Hulst AE, Klip H, Brand PL. Risk of developing asthma in young children with atopic eczema: a systematic review. J Allergy Clin Immunol. 2007;120(3):565–9.
11. Ricci G, Patrizi A, Baldi E, Menna G, Tabanelli M, Masi M. Long-term follow-up of atopic dermatitis: retrospective analysis of related risk factors and association with concomitant allergic diseases. J Am Acad Dermatol. 2006;55(5):765–71.
12. Kapoor R, Menon C, Hoffstad O, Bilker W, Leclerc P, Margolis DJ. The prevalence of atopic triad in children with physician-confirmed atopic dermatitis. J Am Acad Dermatol. 2008;58(1):68–73.
13. Akhouri S, House SA. Allergic rhinitis. StatPearls. Treasure Island (FL): StatPearls Publishing Copyright © 2022, StatPearls Publishing LLC.; 2022.
14. Langan SM, Irvine AD, Weidinger S. Atopic dermatitis. Lancet (British edition). 2020;396(10247):345–60.
15. Alm B, Goksör E, Thengilsdottir H, Pettersson R, Möllborg P, Norvenius G, et al. Early protective and risk factors for allergic rhinitis at age 4½ yr. Pediatr Allergy Immunol. 2011;22(4):398–404.
16. Tran MM, Lefebvre DL, Dharma C, Dai D, Lou WYW, Subbarao P, et al. Predicting the atopic march: results from the Canadian healthy infant longitudinal development study. J Allergy Clin Immunol. 2018;141(2):601–7.e8.
17. Paternoster L, Savenije OEM, Heron J, Evans DM, Vonk JM, Brunekreef B, et al. Identification of atopic dermatitis subgroups in children from 2 longitudinal birth cohorts. J Allergy Clin Immunol. 2018;141(3):964–71.
18. Davis DMR, Drucker AM, Alikhan A, Bercovitch L, Cohen DE, Darr JM, et al. American Academy of Dermatology guidelines: awareness of comorbidities associated with atopic dermatitis in adults. J Am Acad Dermatol. 2022;86(6):1335–6 e18.
19. Lee JH, Son SW, Cho SH. A comprehensive review of the treatment of atopic eczema. Allergy Asthma Immunol Res. 2016;8(3):181–90.
20. Papapostolou N, Xepapadaki P, Gregoriou S, Makris M. Atopic dermatitis and food allergy: a complex interplay what we know and what we would like to learn. J Clin Med. 2022;11(14)
21. Domínguez O, Plaza AM, Alvaro M. Relationship between atopic dermatitis and food allergy. Curr Pediatr Rev. 2020;16(2):115–22.
22. Lack G, Fox D, Northstone K, Golding J. Factors associated with the development of peanut allergy in childhood. N Engl J Med. 2003;348(11):977–85.
23. Brough HA, Nadeau KC, Sindher SB, Alkotob SS, Chan S, Bahnson HT, et al. Epicutaneous sensitization in the development of food allergy: what is the evidence and how can this be prevented? Allergy. 2020;75(9):2185–205.
24. Tham EH, Rajakulendran M, Lee BW, Van Bever HPS. Epicutaneous sensitization to food allergens in atopic dermatitis: what do we know? Pediatr Allergy Immunol. 2020;31(1):7–18.
25. Kim BE, Leung DYM. Significance of skin barrier dysfunction in atopic dermatitis. Allergy Asthma Immunol Res. 2018;10(3):207–15.
26. Alduraywish SA, Lodge CJ, Campbell B, Allen KJ, Erbas B, Lowe AJ, et al. The march from early life food sensitization to allergic disease: a systematic review and meta-analyses of birth cohort studies. Allergy. 2016;71(1):77–89.
27. Yu HS, Tu HP, Hong CH, Lee CH. Lifetime increased risk of adult onset atopic dermatitis in adolescent and adult patients with food allergy. Int J Mol Sci. 2016;18(1)
28. Ben-Shoshan M, Soller L, Harrington DW, Knoll M, La Vieille S, Fragapane J, et al. Eczema in early childhood, sociodemographic factors and lifestyle habits are associated with food allergy: a nested case-control study. Int Arch Allergy Immunol. 2015;166(3):199–207.
29. Martin PE, Eckert JK, Koplin JJ, Lowe AJ, Gurrin LC, Dharmage SC, et al. Which infants with eczema are at risk of food allergy? Results from a population-based cohort. Clin Exp Allergy. 2015;45(1):255–64.

30. Tsakok TMMA, Marrs TMM, Mohsin MMD, Baron SM, Du Toit GF, Till SFP, et al. Does atopic dermatitis cause food allergy? A systematic review. J Allergy Clin Immunol. 2016;137(4):1071–8.
31. Zutavern A, Brockow I, Schaaf B, von Berg A, Diez U, Borte M, et al. Timing of solid food introduction in relation to eczema, asthma, allergic rhinitis, and food and inhalant sensitization at the age of 6 years: results from the prospective birth cohort study LISA. Pediatrics. 2008;121(1):e44–52.
32. Zutavern A, Brockow I, Schaaf B, Bolte G, von Berg A, Diez U, et al. Timing of solid food introduction in relation to atopic dermatitis and atopic sensitization: results from a prospective birth cohort study. Pediatrics. 2006;117(2):401–11.
33. Ho MH, Wong WH, Chang C. Clinical spectrum of food allergies: a comprehensive review. Clin Rev Allergy Immunol. 2014;46(3):225–40.
34. Wassmann A, Werfel T. Atopic eczema and food allergy. Chem Immunol Allergy. 2015;101:181–90.
35. Meyer R, Fox AT, Chebar Lozinsky A, Michaelis LJ, Shah N. Non-IgE-mediated gastrointestinal allergies-do they have a place in a new model of the allergic march. Pediatr Allergy Immunol. 2019;30(2):149–58.
36. Dhar S, Srinivas SM. Food allergy in atopic dermatitis. Indian J Dermatol. 2016;61(6):645–8.
37. Gustafsson D, Sjöberg O, Foucard T. Development of allergies and asthma in infants and young children with atopic dermatitis—a prospective follow-up to 7 years of age. Allergy. 2000;55(3):240–5.
38. Silverberg JI, Gelfand JM, Margolis DJ, Boguniewicz M, Fonacier L, Grayson MH, et al. Association of atopic dermatitis with allergic, autoimmune, and cardiovascular comorbidities in US adults. Ann Allergy Asthma Immunol. 2018;121(5):604–12.e3.
39. Eigenmann PA, Sicherer SH, Borkowski TA, Cohen BA, Sampson HA. Prevalence of IgE-mediated food allergy among children with atopic dermatitis. Pediatrics. 1998;101(3):E8.
40. Cartledge N, Chan S. Atopic dermatitis and food allergy: a paediatric approach. Curr Pediatr Rev. 2018;14(3):171–9.
41. Rancé F. Atopic dermatitis and food allergy: when and how to test. Clin Transl Allergy. 2011;1(S1):S24.
42. Worm M. Atopic dermatitis and food allergy: when and how to test? Clin Transl Allergy. 2011;1(1):S25.
43. Burks AW, James JM, Hiegel A, Wilson G, Wheeler JG, Jones SM, et al. Atopic dermatitis and food hypersensitivity reactions. J Pediatr. 1998;132(1):132–6.
44. Ramírez-Marín HA, Singh AM, Ong PY, Silverberg JI. Food allergy testing in atopic dermatitis. JAAD Int. 2022;9:50–6.
45. Singh AM, Anvari S, Hauk P, Lio P, Nanda A, Sidbury R, et al. Atopic dermatitis and food allergy: best practices and knowledge gaps—a work group report from the AAAAI allergic skin diseases committee and leadership institute project. J Allergy Clin Immunol Pract (Cambridge, MA). 2022;10(3):697–706.
46. Chang A, Robison R, Cai M, Singh AM. Natural history of food-triggered atopic dermatitis and development of immediate reactions in children. J Allergy Clin Immunol Pract. 2016;4(2):229–36.e1.
47. Graham F, Eigenmann PA. Atopic dermatitis and its relation to food allergy. Curr Opin Allergy Clin Immunol. 2020;20(3):305–10.
48. Ridd MJ, Webb D, Roberts K, Santer M, Chalmers JR, Gilbertson A, et al. Test-guided dietary management of eczema in children: a randomized controlled feasibility trial (TEST). Clin Exp Allergy. 2021;51(3):452–62.
49. Batchelor JM, Ridd MJ, Clarke T, Ahmed A, Cox M, Crowe S, et al. The eczema priority setting partnership: a collaboration between patients, carers, clinicians and researchers to identify and prioritize important research questions for the treatment of eczema. Br J Dermatol. 2013;168(3):577–82.
50. Furuta GT, Katzka DA. Eosinophilic esophagitis. N Engl J Med. 2015;373(17):1640–8.

51. Doucet-Ladevèze R, Holvoet S, Raymond F, Foata F, Hershey GKK, Sherrill JD, et al. Transcriptomic analysis links eosinophilic esophagitis and atopic dermatitis. Front Pediatr. 2019;7:467.
52. Assa'ad AHMD, Putnam PEMD, Collins MHMD, Akers RMMPH, Jameson SC, Kirby CL, et al. Pediatric patients with eosinophilic esophagitis: an 8-year follow-up. J Allergy Clin Immunol. 2007;119(3):731–8.
53. Muir A, Falk GW. Eosinophilic esophagitis: a review. JAMA. 2021;326(13):1310–8.
54. Benninger MS, Strohl M, Holy CE, Hanick AL, Bryson PC. Prevalence of atopic disease in patients with eosinophilic esophagitis. Int Forum Allergy Rhinol. 2017;7(8):757–62.
55. Mohammad AA, Wu SZ, Ibrahim O, Bena J, Rizk M, Piliang M, et al. Prevalence of atopic comorbidities in eosinophilic esophagitis: a case-control study of 449 patients. J Am Acad Dermatol. 2017;76(3):559–60.
56. Capucilli P, Cianferoni A, Grundmeier RW, Spergel JM. Comparison of comorbid diagnoses in children with and without eosinophilic esophagitis in a large population. Ann Allergy Asthma Immunol. 2018;121(6):711–6.
57. Daley A, Lehman E, Jhaveri P. Association of initial esophageal eosinophil counts with atopic dermatitis in patients with eosinophilic esophagitis. Ann Allergy Asthma Immunol. 2021;127(6):696–7.
58. Blanchard C, Mingler MK, Vicario M, Abonia JP, Wu YY, Lu TX, et al. IL-13 involvement in eosinophilic esophagitis: transcriptome analysis and reversibility with glucocorticoids. J Allergy Clin Immunol. 2007;120(6):1292–300.
59. Hirano I, Collins MH, Assouline-Dayan Y, Evans L, Gupta S, Schoepfer AM, et al. RPC4046, a monoclonal antibody against IL13, reduces histologic and endoscopic activity in patients with eosinophilic esophagitis. Gastroenterology. 2019;156(3):592–603.e10.
60. Hirano I, Dellon ES, Hamilton JD, Collins MH, Peterson K, Chehade M, et al. Efficacy of dupilumab in a phase 2 randomized trial of adults with active eosinophilic esophagitis. Gastroenterology. 2020;158(1):111–22.e10.
61. Capucilli P, Hill DA. Allergic comorbidity in eosinophilic esophagitis: mechanistic relevance and clinical implications. Clin Rev Allergy Immunol. 2019;57(1):111–27.
62. An SY, Choi HG, Kim SW, Park B, Lee JS, Jang JH, et al. Analysis of various risk factors predisposing subjects to allergic rhinitis. Asian Pac J Allergy Immunol. 2015;33(2):143–51.
63. Hruby A, Hu FB. The epidemiology of obesity: a big picture. PharmacoEconomics. 2015;33(7):673–89.
64. Shan LS, Zhou QL, Shang YX. Bidirectional association between asthma and obesity during childhood and adolescence: a systematic review and meta-analysis. Front Pediatr. 2020;8:576858.
65. Boulet LP. Obesity and atopy. Clin Exp Allergy. 2015;45(1):75–86.
66. Zheng J, Zhang X, Zhang L, Zhang HP, Wang L, Wang G. Interactive effects between obesity and atopy on inflammation: a pilot study for asthma phenotypic overlap. Ann Allergy Asthma Immunol. 2016;117(6):716–7.
67. Ascott A, Mansfield KE, Schonmann Y, Mulick A, Abuabara K, Roberts A, et al. Atopic eczema and obesity: a population-based study. Br J Dermatol (1951). 2021;184(5):871–9.
68. Sybilski AJ, Raciborski F, Lipiec A, Tomaszewska A, Lusawa A, Furmańczyk K, et al. Obesity—a risk factor for asthma, but not for atopic dermatitis, allergic rhinitis and sensitization. Public Health Nutr. 2015;18(3):530–6.
69. Murray CS, Canoy D, Buchan I, Woodcock A, Simpson A, Custovic A. Body mass index in young children and allergic disease: gender differences in a longitudinal study. Clin Exp Allergy. 2011;41(1):78–85.
70. Luo X, Xiang J, Dong X, Cai F, Suo J, Wang Z, et al. Association between obesity and atopic disorders in Chinese adults: an individually matched case-control study. BMC Public Health. 2013;13(1):12.
71. Silverberg JI, Silverberg NB, Lee-Wong M. Association between atopic dermatitis and obesity in adulthood. Br J Dermatol (1951). 2012;166(3):498–504.

72. Silverberg JI, Kleiman E, Lev-Tov H, Silverberg NB, Durkin HG, Joks R, et al. Association between obesity and atopic dermatitis in childhood: a case-control study. J Allergy Clin Immunol. 2011;127(5):1180–6.e1.
73. Van Gysel D, Govaere E, Verhamme K, Doli E, De Baets F. Body mass index in Belgian schoolchildren and its relationship with sensitization and allergic symptoms. Pediatr Allergy Immunol. 2009;20(3):246–53.
74. Tanaka K, Miyake Y, Arakawa M, Sasaki S, Ohya Y. U-shaped association between body mass index and the prevalence of wheeze and asthma, but not eczema or rhinoconjunctivitis: the ryukyus child health study. J Asthma. 2011;48(8):804–10.
75. Oliveira C, Torres T. More than skin deep: the systemic nature of atopic dermatitis. Eur J Dermatol. 2019;29(3):250–8.
76. Epsley S, Tadros S, Farid A, Kargilis D, Mehta S, Rajapakse CS. The effect of inflammation on bone. Front Physiol. 2020;11:511799.
77. Uluçkan Ö, Jimenez M, Karbach S, Jeschke A, Graña O, Keller J, et al. Chronic skin inflammation leads to bone loss by IL-17-mediated inhibition of Wnt signaling in osteoblasts. Sci Transl Med. 2016;8(330):330ra37.
78. Liu T, Li S, Ying S, Tang S, Ding Y, Li Y, et al. The IL-23/IL-17 pathway in inflammatory skin diseases: from bench to bedside. Front Immunol. 2020;11:594735.
79. Bonefeld CM, Petersen TH, Bandier J, Agerbeck C, Linneberg A, Ross-Hansen K, et al. Epidermal filaggrin deficiency mediates increased systemic T-helper 17 immune response. Br J Dermatol (1951). 2016;175(4):706–12.
80. Garg NK, Silverberg JI. Eczema is associated with osteoporosis and fractures in adults: a US population-based study. J Allergy Clin Immunol. 2015;135(4):1085–7.e2.
81. Shaheen MS, Silverberg JI. Atopic dermatitis is associated with osteoporosis and osteopenia in older adults. J Am Acad Dermatol. 2019;80(2):550–1.
82. Wu CY, Lu YY, Lu CC, Su YF, Tsai TH, Wu CH. Osteoporosis in adult patients with atopic dermatitis: a nationwide population-based study. PLoS One. 2017;12(2):e0171667.
83. Wu D, Wu XD, Zhou X, Huang W, Luo C, Liu Y. Bone mineral density, osteopenia, osteoporosis, and fracture risk in patients with atopic dermatitis: a systematic review and meta-analysis. Ann Transl Med. 2021;9(1):40.
84. Lowe KE, Mansfield KE, Delmestri A, Smeeth L, Roberts A, Abuabara K, et al. Atopic eczema and fracture risk in adults: a population-based cohort study. J Allergy Clin Immunol. 2020;145(2):563–71.e8.
85. Garg N, Silverberg JI. Association between eczema and increased fracture and bone or joint injury in adults: a US population-based study. JAMA Dermatol. 2015;151(1):33–41.
86. Haeck IM, Hamdy NA, Timmer-de Mik L, Lentjes EG, Verhaar HJ, Knol MJ, et al. Low bone mineral density in adult patients with moderate to severe atopic dermatitis. Br J Dermatol. 2009;161(6):1248–54.
87. Aalto-Korte K, Turpeinen M. Bone mineral density in patients with atopic dermatitis. Br J Dermatol. 1997;136(2):172–5.
88. Rivers J. Skin inflammation and cardiovascular health. J Cutan Med Surg. 2012;16(5):291–2.
89. Hojman L, Karsulovic C. Cardiovascular disease-associated skin conditions. Vasc Health Risk Manag. 2022;18:43–53.
90. Ascott A, Mulick A, Yu AM, Prieto-Merino D, Schmidt M, Abuabara K, et al. Atopic eczema and major cardiovascular outcomes: a systematic review and meta-analysis of population-based studies. J Allergy Clin Immunol. 2019;143(5):1821–9.
91. Yousaf M, Ayasse M, Ahmed A, Gwillim EC, Janmohamed SR, Yousaf A, et al. Association between atopic dermatitis and hypertension: a systematic review and meta-analysis. Br J Dermatol (1951). 2022;186(2):227–235.
92. Drucker AM, Harvey PJ. Atopic dermatitis and cardiovascular disease: what are the clinical implications? J Allergy Clin Immunol. 2019;143(5):1736–8.

93. Maintz L, Bieber T, Simpson HD, Demessant-Flavigny AL. From skin barrier dysfunction to systemic impact of atopic dermatitis: implications for a precision approach in dermocosmetics and medicine. J Pers Med. 2022;12(6)
94. Yang G, Seok JK, Kang HC, Cho YY, Lee HS, Lee JY. Skin barrier abnormalities and immune dysfunction in atopic dermatitis. Int J Mol Sci. 2020;21(8)
95. Ivert LU, Wahlgren CF, Lindelöf B, Dal H, Bradley M, Johansson EK. Association between atopic dermatitis and autoimmune diseases: a population-based case-control study. Br J Dermatol. 2021;185(2):335–42.

# Index




N. Brownstone et al. (eds.), *Clinical Cases in Atopic Dermatitis*, Clinical Cases in Dermatology, https://doi.org/10.1007/978-3-031-52147-8

MIX
Papier aus verantwortungsvollen Quellen
Paper from responsible sources
FSC® C105338

If you have any concerns about our products,
you can contact us on
**ProductSafety@springernature.com**

In case Publisher is established outside the EU,
the EU authorized representative is:
**Springer Nature Customer Service Center GmbH**
**Europaplatz 3, 69115 Heidelberg, Germany**

Printed by Libri Plureos GmbH
in Hamburg, Germany